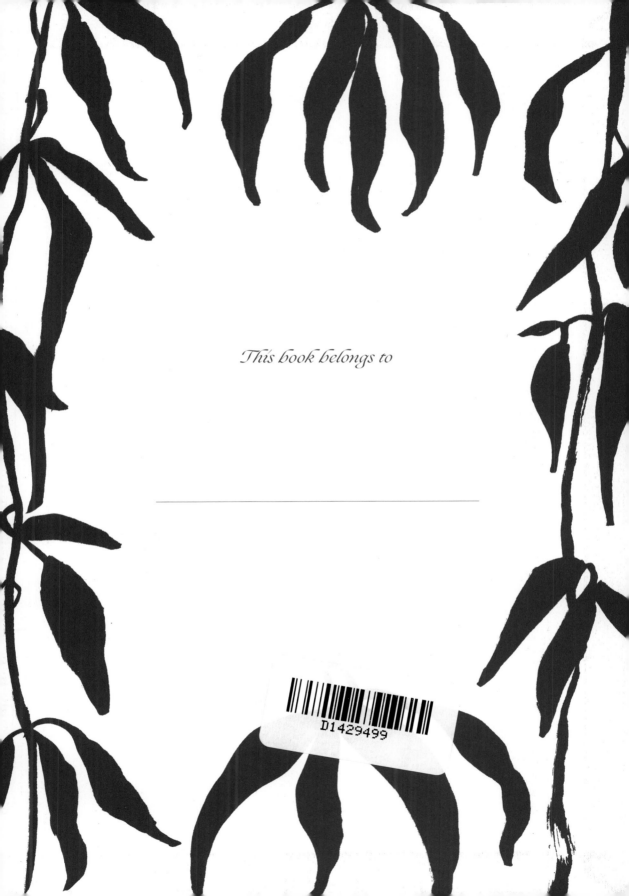

This book belongs to

_____

D1429499

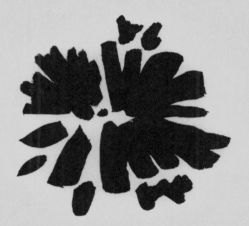

To our daughters, Hannah and Sarah:
the unconditional love we share is beyond words.

Special dedication to Dr Daniel Friedland.
Mentor to both authors.
Pioneer in integrative medicine, major contributor to the
wellness industry and visionary in Conscious Leadership.

Beyond his extraordinary intellect, his capacity for human
connection was beyond exception.

Remembered with gratitude and love.

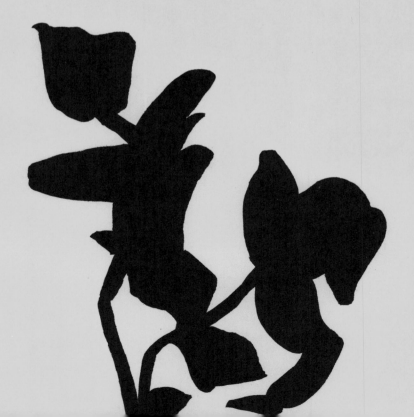

How to Be Well

A Handbook for Women

DR KAREN COATES & SHARON KOLKKA

A JULIE GIBBS BOOK

for

SIMON &
SCHUSTER

London · New York · Sydney · Toronto · New Delhi

TABLE OF CONTENTS

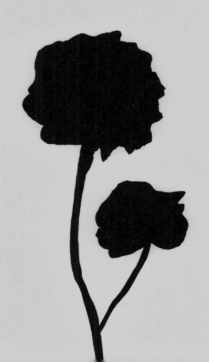

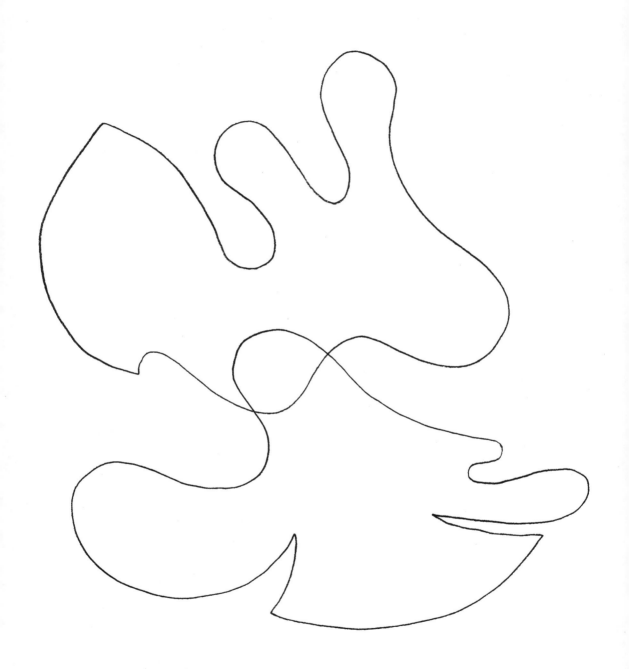

ABOUT THE AUTHORS

DR KAREN COATES

As medical advisor to some of Australia's highest-profile celebrities and elite athletes, Dr. Karen draws on her extensive experience as an integrative medicine doctor and qualifications in surgery, obstetrics, nutritional and environmental medicine. Over her 30-year career she has cared for women of all ages who have come to her with diverse medical challenges. A keen researcher who keeps her finger on the pulse of cutting-edge medicine, Dr Karen is respected for her holistic approach to healthcare which extends beyond the traditional medical model while remaining evidence-based.

Nationally recognised for her expertise in women's health, Karen writes regularly for the mainstream media, sharing her insights, expertise, and opinion on the state of women's health in the 21st Century. She is a sought-after expert in the nutritional arena for programs such as *Today Tonight* and *A Current Affair*.

An advocate for self-responsibility in health, she has a passion for teaching and a gift for explaining complex health concepts in easy-to-understand terminology. She is a published author of *Embracing the Warrior - an Essential Guide for Women*, and mother of Hannah and Michael.

Now retired from clinical work, Karen continues to educate women worldwide on the subject of health, stress, and hormones, teaching them how to manifest wellness from puberty through to the post-menopausal years.

SHARON KOLKKA

Inspiring men and women around Australia to take control of their health and wellness for over 40 years, Sharon Kolkka is one of Australia's leading wellness advisors. Her innovative approach to wellbeing shaped the highly successful and transformative programs at Gwinganna Lifestyle Retreat where she previously held the position of General Manager and Wellness Director for 16 years. A trailblazer in the field of wellness and stress resilience, Sharon has helped to change and transform the lives of tens of thousands of people.

A renowned thought leader, educator and wellness program designer to many progressive retreats and businesses, Sharon is also highly regarded as an international keynote speaker. Regularly featured within the press for her insights into health, wellness and work/life balance, she is passionate about sharing wellness wisdom, helping both men and women to reframe their perspective and cultivate greater stress resilience.

Sharon feels incredibly blessed to be a mum to Sarah, Mum-in-Law to Phil and Grandmother or 'Jams' to Archer James. For Sharon, her family are 'the loves of her life'.

INTRODUCTION

Are you 'overtired, overstretched and over it'?

I've spent more than 30 years in private practice as an integrative medical doctor and I have heard some variation of these words too many times from my patients. And through all those years of private practice, I have taught my patients that there's no need to feel like this. Welcome to *How to Be Well*, where we will teach you why you don't need to feel stressed, exhausted or lacking in joy. My patients have learned they don't have to feel like this. *How to Be Well* is your guide to learning how to live your best life – all day, every day.

In the first few years of my career, my heart would sink when I'd welcome a new patient and, when asking them why they had come to see me, the reply was: 'I'm tired and I don't know why'. I suspect that many doctors slide into indifference when an exhausted patient's basic screening tests for thyroid and iron levels come back within normal range. My approach has been to secretly grin with excitement and say to those women 'Yes! I can help you with that'.

Before making their way to my office, many of my patients had become so despondent with the way they felt, they had turned to 'Dr. Google' to find answers. Cyberspace can be a dangerous and often confusing territory, particularly for those feeling vulnerable and fragile about their health. Many of my patients were desperate to find some solutions, trying to find the first step to take. Thankfully, with some savvy investigation and planning alongside an integrative doctor such as myself, many of those tired and frustrated women are now on a solid wellness path with solutions and ongoing support.

As a passionate medical doctor, I become frustrated with this exhaustion endemic. In Australia, we have a world-class medical system, yet many medical professionals struggle to find time to provide advice for wellness due to the overwhelming demands of looking after the very sick. Time and time again I hear stories from women who are depleted and struggling, looking for advice on how to reconnect with the energy and wellness that they had enjoyed when they were younger. I have come to understand the solutions are rarely found in a doctor's office.

And so, frustrated, these tired, struggling women turn elsewhere – mostly to the internet. Online there are a plethora of wellness transformation programs that claim to heal or fix nearly anything. Unfortunately, many of these programs are offered by people who have had little, if any, training or experience in the health, wellness or medical fields. For people who feel lost and are looking for the answer to their health challenge, it can feel like a miracle to see hundreds of testimonials preaching guaranteed success. And when you've ventured down the medical route to no avail, you think: 'Why not try this? What have I got to lose?'. The answer? Quite a lot.

Sadly, many of these 'gurus' do not have the training to offer clients – women in need of an answer – the big picture. There are innumerable, intricately linked daily processes within our anciently designed body. Many 'motivators' fail to understand that exercise in itself can be a physical stress that can do **both** good and harm. Too much exercise can domino, creating a time bomb of potential health problems that may not reveal themselves for another 10-15 years. By which time it becomes even more difficult to right the wrongs.

What works for one person – guru or not – is not likely to work for another. This is apparent when we consider the emerging evidence from genetic research. Any health and fitness 'guru' who recommends a restrictive eating program or exhaustive exercise regime as a quick fix for your health problems are often failing to understand the complexities of the human body. And how unique our biochemistry is. This information is only available through proper medical channels and assessment.

This book is aimed at these gurus, too - in the hope that when they offer advice to women in need of support, they have a wider sense of what goes into understanding and supporting a woman's health journey.

How to Be Well is a labour of love and a collaboration with my friend and colleague of more than 20 years, Sharon Kolkka. It has been born out of our joint intention to offer solid preventative health care information to those who are either looking for answers on how to improve the way they feel, or those who want to take a preventative approach to their wellness. At the core of our advice sits principles that are based on our combined 70 years of experience in the wellness industry. We have consulted with experts; we have researched papers on health and disease published in respected medical journals; and we are ideally placed to consider both evidence-based conventional medicine along with traditional healing systems.

Most importantly as two women living in the modern world, we also share experiences from our own personal healing journeys.

We hope this book is an invaluable resource in your health and wellness journey.

Welcome aboard.

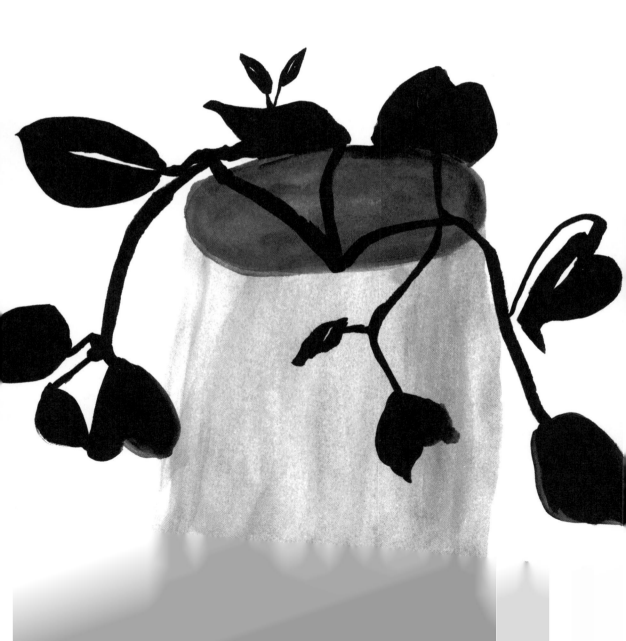

FROM SHARON KOLKKA

With such incredible progressions in the medical industry, why is it that so many of us spend our days feeling exhausted, overwhelmed, stressed and run down?

Having assisted tens of thousands of men and women throughout my career, I am deeply concerned there are still many stories left untold, and solutions that have not yet been presented.

As women, do we feel empowered to take our health into our own hands with evidence-based guidance? Or are we allowing our lifestyle choices to impact how we feel each day? Many of us say we eat well and exercise, yet we still feel exhausted by life in general. Why? After talking with so many women during the last 30 years, I have seen a common thread that binds us; we have an immense drive to get things done. And it's unrelenting.

Without a doubt, women are extraordinary and have an immense capacity to keep all the balls in the air. We take care of family and friends (more often than not whilst still working full time); we want to feel needed, engaged and loved; we want to, and many have to, contribute to the family financially; we want to live life with passion and purpose; or we need to contribute to society in some way. All these goals and pursuits are noble and encouraged, yet there's no denying that there's a mental, emotional and physical fallout. Now is the time to ask, at what cost?

As women, let's gather together and share our collective and authentic wellness wisdom. Not the fads or the quick fixes, but the old-fashioned tried-and-tested, along with the emerging new sciences. Let's empower ourselves to continue to contribute to loved ones and society to get things done – to truly live a vital life. We are amazing, capable and incredible carers with 'to do' and 'to be' lists. There's no escaping these lists - they will still feature in our lives. We hope to share with you that these lists are not the enemy, there is a way you can still tick all the boxes and not break yourself in the process. So that you thrive each day, rather than reaching the end of it exhausted.

Write this on the fridge, or in your diary:

'If I break, everything around me breaks with me'.

As you dig deeper into *How to Be Well* you will realise just why it's so important to put yourself and your health first. Because it's not just about you, it's about your children too. Although common, constant 'busy and stressed' is not a healthy nor natural State of Being.

A stressed body and mind is not living a vital life; it is an existence in a constant state of survival. This state depletes us, it consumes and bleeds the very life out of us. This more than anything contributes to our depletion and is the first step on the road to a disease.

In one way or another, I've been immersed in the wellness industry for most of my adult life. I started in the fitness industry in 1980 and moved into the world of health retreats in 1995. I have always been a researcher and interested in exposing hidden facts about wellbeing. Since I began, my passion and motivation has always been to use my knowledge to inspire and empower those I have the privilege to take care of and to influence them to prioritise their health.

These days, there is so much confusion about what to do in order to be well. Wellness is discussed in so many forums, but not always by those who have the latest in evidence-based research. Unfortunately, in our world of technology with so much at our fingertips, information can become watered down and misinterpreted.

In 2004 I became involved in creating a fully-immersive wellness experience, Gwinganna Lifestyle Retreat, with founder and owner Tony de Leede. When you visit Gwinganna you have access to the latest research and the opportunity to ask questions and experience all aspects of wellness for yourself. However, attending a wellness retreat isn't accessible for all. Hence my desire to share the 40 years of valuable insights I've obtained in the wellness industry in a book.

I have also been lucky enough through my career to meet and get to know incredibly gifted practitioners and researchers, many of whom I now call friends. As a result, the information that I have at my fingertips about evidenced-based, preventative healthcare strategies is staggering. Sadly, we all hear stories about someone who has put their faith into the standard system only to have had it fail them for some reason or another. Western medicine is extraordinary in so many ways, yet it is overwhelmed. As Dr Karen Coates suggests, there's little scope for the recommendation of preventative practices. Sometimes the prevention of a potential problem is the most important element.

Unless we seek relevant information on how to reach and maintain optimal wellness, we can find ourselves fighting health fires that have already been burning for some time, instead of preventing them from igniting in the first place.

More than 20 years ago I heard about an integrative doctor, who was tucked quietly away in the Currumbin Valley working from her home. It took me six months to get in to see Dr Karen Coates! I was sceptical that a doctor could see past a pharmaceutical solution, but I was mistaken. My first consultation with Karen lasted an hour and was like no other doctor visit I had ever experienced. What I found was an extraordinary human, highly intelligent and passionate about research, with her medical hat firmly in place. To my elation (and astonishment) she had also explored complementary medicine, and presented it with a great deal of common sense. From that moment on we became friends. My goal has always been to provide evidence-based advice, backed up by solid research. Dr Karen - the research bunny - delivered every time, and she still does every day.

To share this book-writing journey with her has been a gift. We have laughed, groaned and gasped in shock at some of the research. This book is dedicated to all those who need the information in its pages. It is also a gift for all women who do not have a doctor like Karen.

This book is for women of all ages. Share it, give it, refer to it often. Our purpose and reason for writing this is for you, your friends and family. We want you to be well, healthy and happy. To live your life with vitality and joy with healthy generations to come.

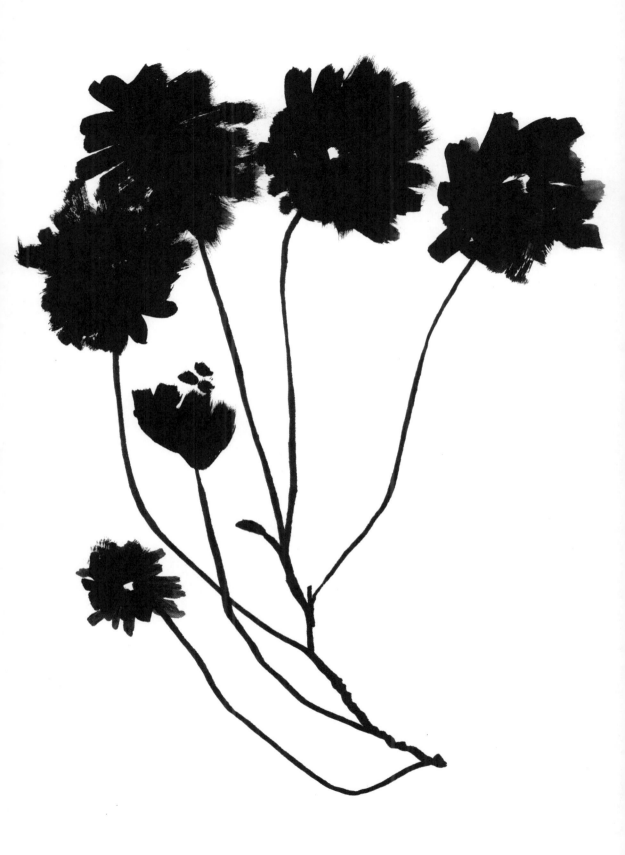

How to
USE THIS BOOK FOR OPTIMAL WELLNESS

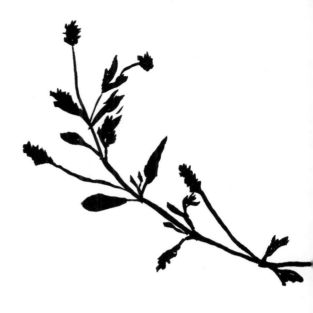

This book is going to become your new best friend, your reference guide, your journal and all round reassurance that you are on the right path for you. We want you to keep it close, refer to it as often as possible, or as necessary, whether it's to reassure yourself, find out more, or follow the daily health and wellness guide at the end of the book.

Remember, each and every one of us is on our own personal journey. No two people's road to wellness is the same. This book is your personal compass to finding out how you can feel the best version of yourself *every single day*.

We invite you to use highlighters, make notes relevant to your unique circumstances and diarise your progress. Continue to revisit the relevant chapters as you progress through the solutions we have outlined in each chapter for you and your family.

Today is the first day of the rest of your life.

WHERE TO GO FROM HERE

Now is the time to find your personal starting point on your lifelong wellness journey. Be sure to take the time to really honour your health. You can do this by finding some space to assess your current State of Being. Then you'll be able to follow these steps to success.

STEP 1

Read through **Chapter 1** and familiarise yourself with the **Three States of Being**. This is your starting point for your health journey and will provide relevance to your unique needs.

STEP 2

Read about the **Five Pillars of Wellness (see page 41)**.

STEP 3

Complete your **Personal Health Audit (see page 52)** and keep a copy of your baseline results for future reference.

STEP 4

Continue to work your way through each chapter. Each chapter contains information relevant to your **current State of Being** and solutions to give you more information to move forward.

STEP 5

At the end of each section work through the **Solutions** and mark those that resonate and are relevant to your unique circumstances.

STEP 6

Make a commitment to the necessary long-term changes in order to achieve your short-term goals.

IMPORTANT NOTE!

As women, it's our natural state to be hard on ourselves. Remember, this book is not about judgement. Rather, it's about honouring your mind, body and spirit, to make the most of your true self every single day.

Be realistic when setting yourself goals. When making changes to your lifestyle, avoid raising the bar too high; be realistic, to ensure your success. Remind yourself to focus on making small changes with a big commitment. This way you'll be continually moving towards better health. No matter where your starting point is, aim for a series of achievable short-term goals and congratulate yourself for every single win.

Commit to a maximum of three tasks at a time and cement those changes over a few weeks before moving on to the next.

For some, this may be a commitment to get off the couch and move for just 10 minutes a day. For others, it may be a commitment to give up two spin classes a week and replace them with a more gentle and restorative movement activity. For others, perhaps they'll commit to drinking sufficient water and eating more plant-based foods.

This is *your* amazing life, live it well.

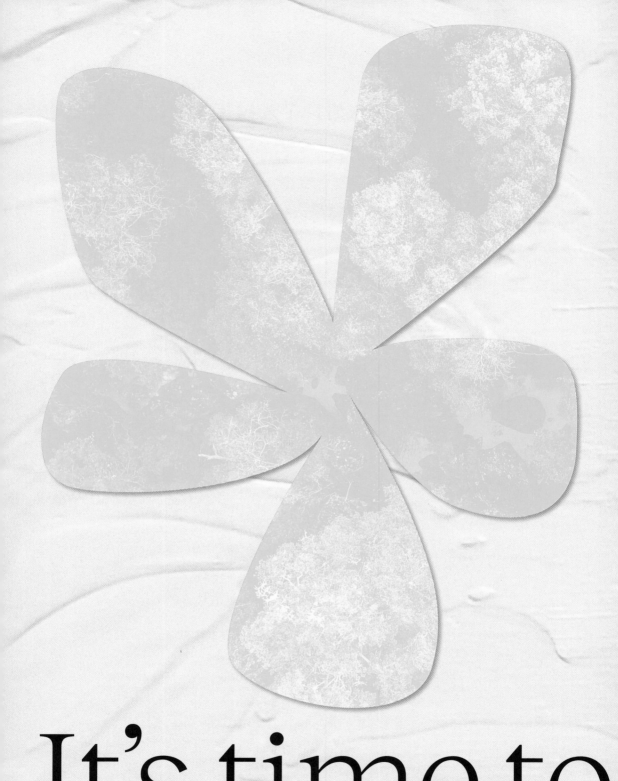

It's time to

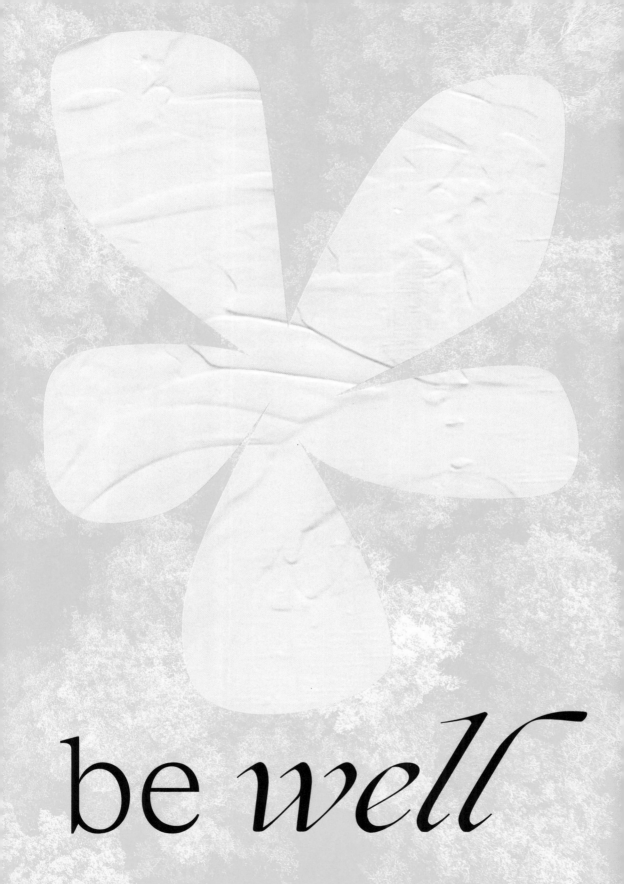

be well

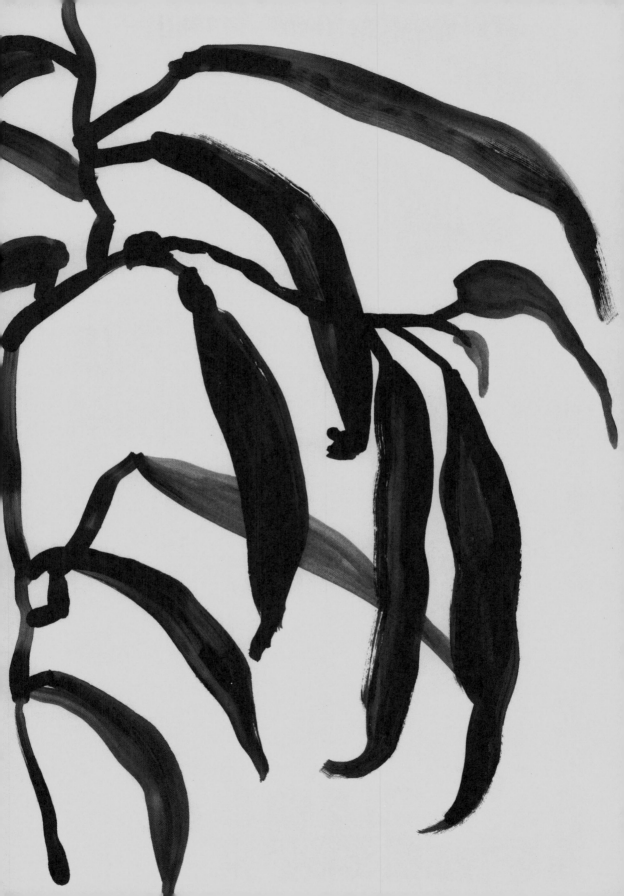

1.
THE THREE
STATES OF BEING

Being:

the quality or state of
having existence.

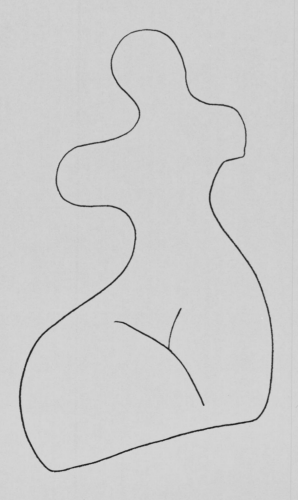

Before we begin, let's take a moment.

We want you to stop and ask yourself:

How do you feel right now?

Are you well?

Happy?

Sad?

Stressed?

Exhausted?

In pain?

Just existing?

How we feel physically and mentally is intrinsically linked: if you're tired, then you're unlikely to be able to deal with stressful situations: if you're happy you're more able to juggle several balls in the air without breaking a sweat.

How you feel each day typically changes (even hour by hour). This is because your body is a living, breathing biological organism. Our bodies are a wonderful thing – they're self-repairing and will age gracefully if treated with respect. They need to be nurtured and offered all the elements that are required for self-maintenance. If we don't take the best care of our physical, mental and emotional health, the wheels begin to fall off and this is when a descent into discomfort, illness or disease can occur (just think about the last time you fell ill – we bet it was after a prolonged stressful or emotionally upsetting period).

Being present and being the best you can be, could help you prevent illness or disease.

Most of us are in one of three **States of Being: Thriving, Surviving,** or **Depleted**. Read through each State of Being on the following pages to find out which one resonates with you.

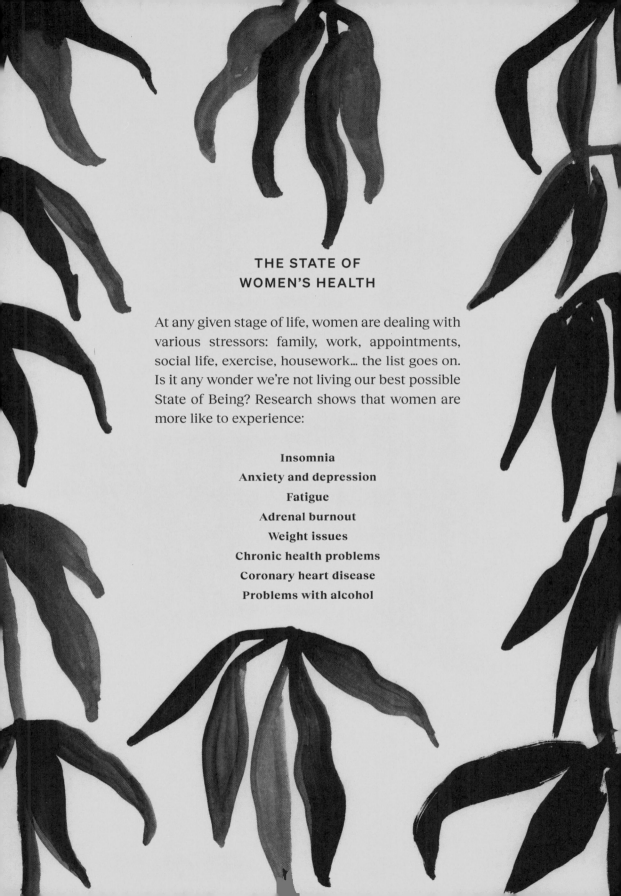

THE STATE OF WOMEN'S HEALTH

At any given stage of life, women are dealing with various stressors: family, work, appointments, social life, exercise, housework... the list goes on. Is it any wonder we're not living our best possible State of Being? Research shows that women are more like to experience:

Insomnia
Anxiety and depression
Fatigue
Adrenal burnout
Weight issues
Chronic health problems
Coronary heart disease
Problems with alcohol

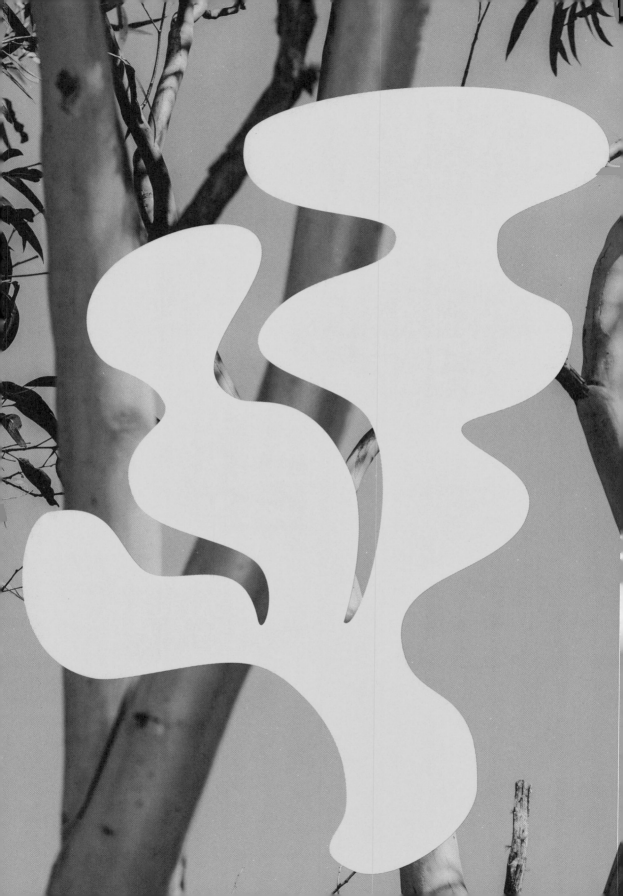

STATE ONE

Thriving

In this state you are living your life with purpose and meaning. Your typical day involves waking up and feeling refreshed from a good seven to eight hours of sleep. Your first thoughts are positive and you are optimistically looking forward to the day's events. As you get out of bed you can feel your energy levels rise.

You love to eat a nourishing wholefood diet and look forward to doing some gentle and dynamic exercise. You know that giving energy to yourself before you give to others feels right, and you love this 'me time' in your day. This self-care allows you to take care of others with energy and love, without resentment.

During the day you have energy to meet obstacles if and when they arise. You feel open and accepting that sometimes things might not go your way. You feel relaxed, patient and tolerant, with a capacity to acknowledge and accept that others may not be in the same state of thriving as you are.

This is me! Can I pat myself on the back?

This glorious State of Being feels as though your life is in flow, where it's easy to find joy and happiness in most situations. However, this does not mean your wellness journey is done! It's important to remain acutely aware that you still need to monitor and make any necessary adjustments to your lifestyle to sustain the ideal equilibrium and good health.

STATE TWO

Surviving

We suspect many women fall into this category: you're not unwell, nor are you leaping out of bed with energy and enthusiasm each morning. You don't have any particular symptoms, but you also know that you're not as healthy as you could be. You often feel wired but tired, and you know that something has to change. But who has the time to investigate when there is so much to keep on top of? You fear that if you stop you will lose the plot, become overwhelmed and under-achieving, and you are not sure you could pick it all up again. You can keep going, provided you are stimulated with caffeine, sugar, exercise or pressure. The truth is you are more tired and exhausted than you are willing to admit. Your eating and exercise habits are probably inconsistent, and there are some days you're relatively healthy, and other days where you fall off the wagon.

This State of Being means you are not being particularly present within your life. Fuelled by caffeine, sugar and stress, you lurch from one task or stressful situation to another.

This is me! How can I improve my State of Being?

While this State of Being is maintainable for the moment, long-term you will find that you'll no longer be able to recover as quickly from a weekend of overeating and drinking, or from sleepless nights or stressful situations. This is the perfect time to address your life balance.

STATE THREE

Depleted

You probably feel as though you have hit rock bottom. Whether mentally, emotionally and/or physically, you are in a state of depletion. You lack energy from the moment you open your eyes in the morning (and even that is an effort!). A good night's sleep is rare. As a consequence, everything feels difficult, as though the smallest of tasks requires superhuman effort. At times you wonder if you will ever feel different and have energy once more.

This lack of energy affects your daily outlook and your inner-voice may be incredibly self-critical. You may feel overwhelmed and unsupported by the people in your life. There seems to be too much to do and so little energy available to get it done. Perhaps life circumstances have prevented self-care from being a priority for you, due to stress, work or various life factors, such as a devastating emotional blow, a critical medical diagnosis or an accident (or perhaps all of the above). You may feel overwhelmed and wonder if you will ever feel really well again.

This is me! SOS!

If this is your State of Being, it's time to begin your journey towards better health. The journey may be confronting and at times you may feel like giving up, and returning to the more stressful but familiar depleted state. Be brave, you are stronger than you think. We've got you.

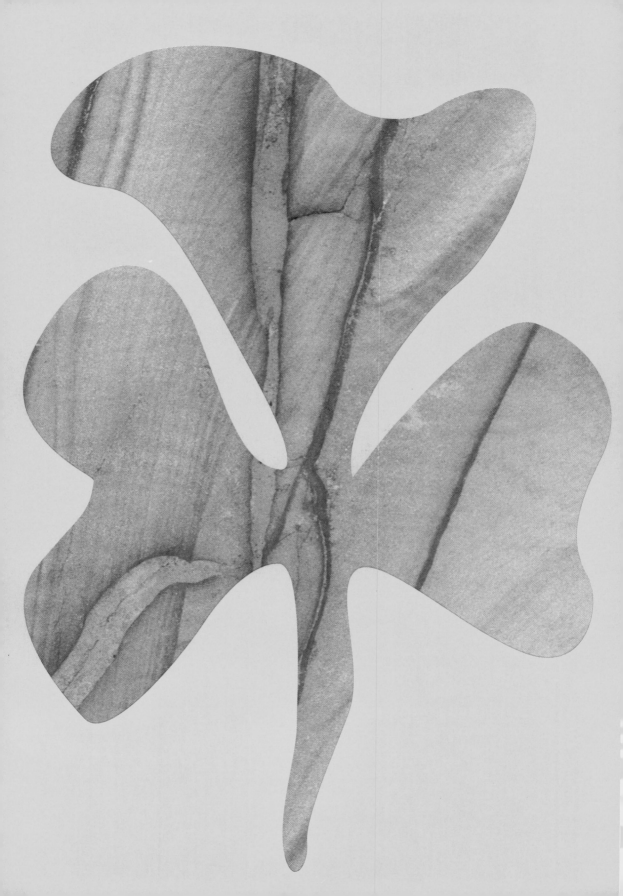

What now?

Identifying with one of the three **States of Being** is your first step towards better health: physically, emotionally and mentally. Each stage provides its own set of challenges for your wellness journey and requires a different plan of action.

As you read on you will see that we have provided strategies for your specific State of Being (Thriving, Surviving or Depleted).

Those who are Thriving
need to maintain the positive balance found in this state.

Those who are Surviving
need to work on the foundations of wellness that are
lacking in their busy life.

For those who are Depleted,
take a big breath. You will have a longer road ahead of you,
so it's imperative that you are willing to develop new lifestyle habits that
support health. We will start you with tiny steps, each of which is bathed
in self-compassion and self-care.

MOVING FROM DEPLETED TO SURVIVING…
TO THRIVING

The **Recommendations** within each chapter allow you to develop and implement the right strategies to move your health towards a thriving state of wellness. At the end of each chapter you will find **Solutions** to help you. Revisit these wellness messages and solutions to ensure you stay on the right wellness path for your life. Take note of the icons which identify important information for each State of Being.

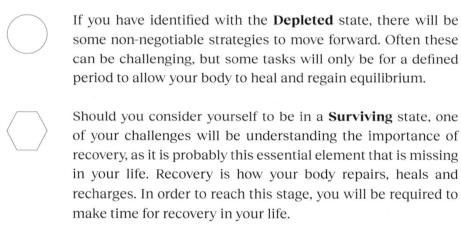

If you have identified with the **Depleted** state, there will be some non-negotiable strategies to move forward. Often these can be challenging, but some tasks will only be for a defined period to allow your body to heal and regain equilibrium.

Should you consider yourself to be in a **Surviving** state, one of your challenges will be understanding the importance of recovery, as it is probably this essential element that is missing in your life. Recovery is how your body repairs, heals and recharges. In order to reach this stage, you will be required to make time for recovery in your life.

Once you reach your **Thriving** state, it's important not to rest on your laurels. You will still need to monitor and manage your lifestyle to maintain this ultimate expression of health and wellness. Keep this book close if a health challenge presents.

Our aim is to help you thrive and to assist you, in times of need, to regain your momentum towards living a long, happy and healthy life.

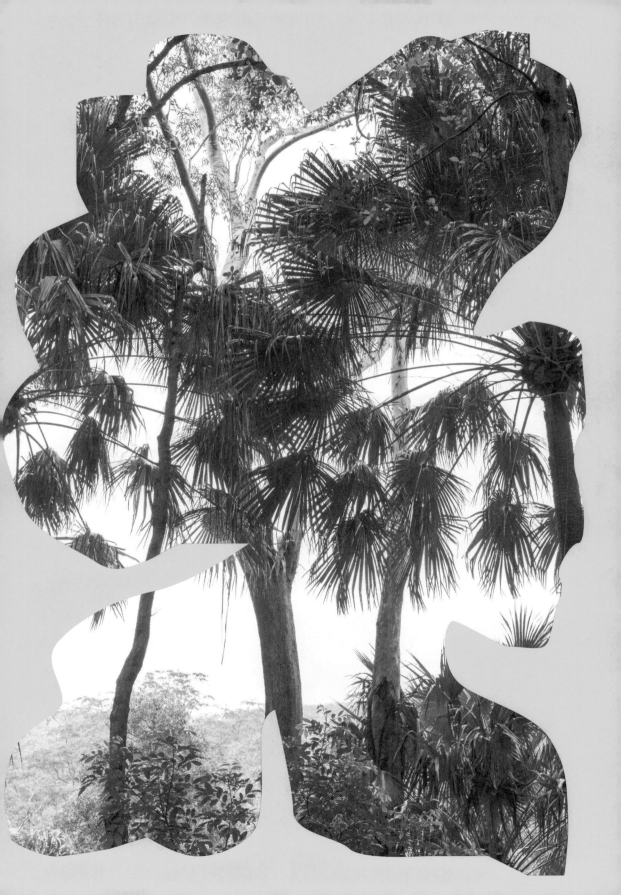

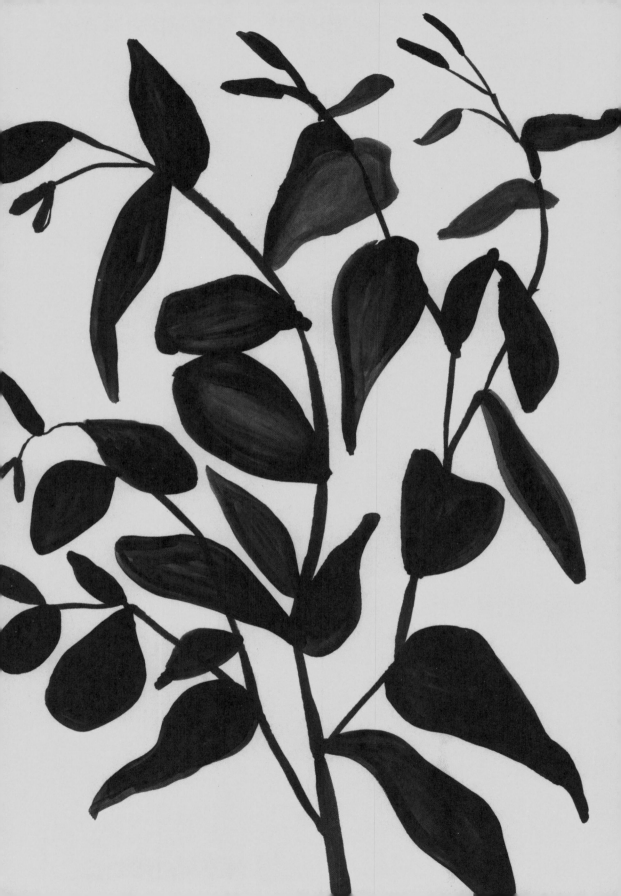

2.
THE FIVE PILLARS OF WELLNESS

Pillar One
NOURISHMENT

Pillar Two
FUNCTIONAL MOVEMENT

Pillar Three
EMOTIONAL WELLBEING AND STRESS RESILIENCE

Pillar Four
SLEEP

Pillar Five
THRIVING IN A FAST-PACED AND TOXIC WORLD

The part can never be well unless the whole is well.

PLATO

WHAT IS YOUR CIRCADIAN RHYTHM?

This is our natural internal body clock that is reset by light and darkness every 24 hours. This clock operates our sleep-wake cycle and is the master control that ensures our natural biochemical processes operate in perfect alignment for optimal wellbeing.

If you believe in the theory of evolution, scientifically speaking the human body has evolved very little over the past 40 thousand years. In stark contrast, our physical and social environment has undergone many immense changes.

Some scientists theorise that our body responds best to the things we are 'naturally' designed to do, such as following the body's circadian rhythm, squatting on our haunches every day, walking, being in nature, resting and eating a plant-based diet. However, what is 'natural' for our species is very different from what has become the 'normal' way we expect our bodies to live and exist in today's world. We need to redefine 'normal'.

We spend more than 100 days online every year.

It may be 'normal' for us to check social media and browse the internet into the late evening, but this cannot be considered 'natural'. Sitting in a chair all day long is something we are not designed to do, biologically speaking – it's not 'natural' and yet it is a very 'normal' part of our lives today.

So how do we define the difference between 'natural' and 'normal'? The difference between the two is the health problems or issues that arise due to our lack of 'natural' living. Think of them as the grit of sand in the oyster – but in this case, a pearl isn't created! This irritation creates disharmony in our cells, interferes with our circadian rhythm and our sleep, or disrupts the nutritional needs of our body. In other words, doing things we accept as 'normal' in our everyday life can lead to imbalances in our body.

Throughout the rest of this book you'll find tips and solutions that will support the following **Five Pillars of Wellness** to ensure you feel and look your best throughout all stages of your life.

THE FIVE PILLARS OF WELLNESS

These five pillars work concurrently to ensure that you are living in optimum health with a balanced physical, mental and emotional state. When one or more of the five key pillars are out of balance, you can experience discomfort, pain or illness that affects the quality of your life.

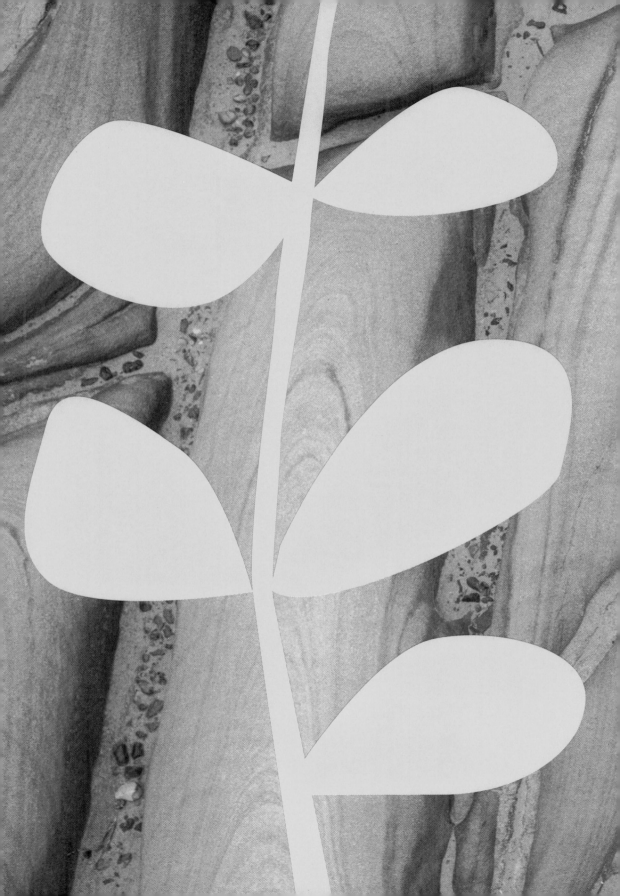

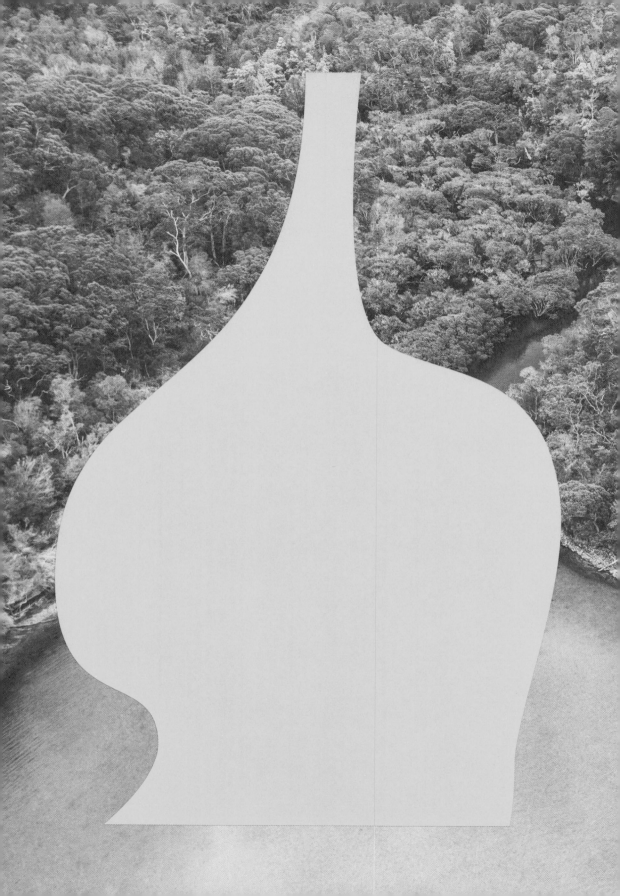

PILLAR ONE

Nourishment

When we consider nourishment, we're talking about how well your body is nourished on a cellular level. This starts with the food you eat and how well you digest it, whether the nutrients are absorbed from your gut, reaching the cells in your body, and the overall quality of your food. The food you're eating may be healthy, but is it good for *you specifically*? Not always. There is no one size fits all for all sorts of reasons. Heritage can influence food intolerances. For example, if you are of Asian descent, you may have sensitivity to dairy as these foods have not been a part of your ancestral diet. Similarly, grains were not a huge part of the ancestral diet in Ireland and so many people with Irish heritage have a gluten intolerance. Many First Nations peoples have difficulty processing sugar (in all its forms) and have a higher risk of diabetes, because their diet for thousands of years was so incredibly pure. Additionally, many commercially grown foods may contain or have traces of toxins and chemicals which may impede or impact your ability to nourish the 50 trillion cells in your body.

PILLAR TWO

Functional movement

Having healthy functional movement means the ability to retain independence well into your older years, as you avoid bone degeneration, stiffness and inflammatory problems that can impede your range of motion.

Our bodies respond to movement on an ancient, hardwired template. Human beings are designed to walk, run, squat, lunge, push and pull things and rotate our spine. As a species, we also seem to be hardwired to music. Have you ever noticed how your foot may tap when you hear your favourite song, or maybe you spontaneously dance to the beat of the music? Maintaining these functions involves an intricate dance between muscle, bone, the nervous system and brain. Posture, your basal metabolic rate (the energy you expend when resting), and your ability to maintain a healthy body weight also all come into play. If this dance is in perfect balance, all these elements work together to allow you pain-free movement.

The way you choose to move feeds information about your environment through the nervous system back and forth to the midbrain. These messages control your biochemistry. Get the balance of movement right and you will thrive. Get it wrong and the domino effect activates stress pathways that interfere with the way your body functions in everyday life.

Here's one example. Sitting switches off your core muscles, tightens your hip flexor muscles and disrupts your posture. This pulls the body's equilibrium out of balance, like a tent pole that is crooked because the ropes are pulled tighter on one side. Some symptoms from imbalances in your muscular system may include back pain, neck pain and headaches.

PILLAR THREE

Emotional wellbeing and stress resilience

How happy you are, how you deal with pressure and how you process sad or anxious situations depends on your emotional wellbeing. This complex area of wellness can often be neglected by mainstream medicine, as it is common for this modality to treat the symptom rather than addressing the deeper cause.

The connection between emotional and physical wellbeing is hard to dissect. Both emotional and physical wellness are connected via the brain and nervous system. Your emotional wellbeing affects all your biochemical pathways and influences how you feel about your life and your place within it. Without a strong foundational emotional balance, your ability to manage stressful situations will be compromised.

We like to use the 'bucket of water' system. If your emotional wellbeing is balanced, your bucket is full. If a stressful situation arises, then you have water in your bucket to put out that fire. If your bucket is empty though, or doesn't get refilled, that stressful situation becomes magnified.

Whether you identify with being stressed or not, the reality is the pace of the modern world is activating your ancient stress response. Advances in technology have resulted in unprecedented psychological and social stimulants at levels that far exceed anything we've been exposed to before in human history. By being 'plugged in' almost all the time, with huge expectations on yourself and others, life moves faster than ever, with little or no downtime.

Since Covid-19 has entered the world, the baseline level of psychological and psychosocial stress has skyrocketed. Alongside a pandemic, society has, and is facing, a mental and emotional health crisis. Your ability to navigate the perceptions created by your beliefs and experiences has never been more important. The expectations to disseminate information, news, world events and social or family demands can be overwhelming. For some, the 'ting' of a message creates a Pavlovian response: to do, to act, to reply. There is a different way to approach life, one that allows you the freedom to enjoy the present moment and reduce feelings of pressure and overwhelm.

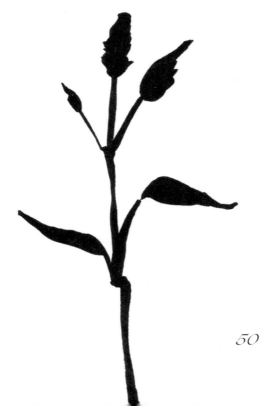

PILLAR FOUR

Sleep

This pillar is non-negotiable: sleep. Ask any new mum, busy mum, working woman, or just any woman – if they get enough sleep. Most likely, the answer will be, 'No!' (or something less polite).

Sleep is not a luxury. Sleep is a necessity! Yet, lack of quality sleep is a modern-day plague that stems from overstimulation, technology, artificial lighting and an increasingly fast-paced way of living. Without sleep your body cannot repair cells, detoxify itself or function well. What does this mean? Without long-term quality sleep you will be more susceptible to stress and disease, fat gain, not to mention the inability to make well-balanced decisions for your health as you may continue the cycle of reaching for caffeine and sugar in order to power your way through the day.

It's time to prioritise good sleep habits.

Until you take the appropriate action to improve your sleep, increased vitality and optimal wellness will be an elusive dream.

Did you know that the hormonal changes of breastfeeding are designed to protect new mothers from the negative effects of sleep disruption?

MORE IN CHAPTER 9 (SEE PAGE 334)

YOUR PERSONAL HEALTH AUDIT

Before you read through the chapters detailing the Five Pillars, complete your personal audit. You don't need to share this with anyone, nor is anybody judging your answers. These are for your eyes only. You may find that you're strong in some pillars, and not as strong or focused on others. The idea is to find out which areas need work, and which areas may be allowed to rest in the background while you do so.

Now is the time to be scrupulously honest with yourself about the way things really are. Only from here can you begin to take the actions that will lead to the wonderful changes you are looking for.

Change is good.

When it comes to making health or lifestyle changes, it's typical to gravitate towards things or situations you feel comfortable with, and avoid ones which are uncomfortable or too challenging. You may find that tackling those areas you resist the most will result in the biggest reward. So, take a deep breath, sit down with a cup of herbal tea. It's time to find out how you are going to live a happier and healthier life.

There may be a difference between the person you present to the world compared to behind the scenes, and what you are truly experiencing, or thinking. Perhaps you don't want to be a burden, you don't want to let people down, or don't want to be perceived as a failure. So instead, you may present an image or 'window dressing' of what's really going on behind a brave face. Perhaps, since we have all faced a Covid-19 crisis, it's now time to be really honest about what is going on and unpack the true state of your physical, mental and emotional wellbeing.

Create a life that feels good on the inside, not one that just looks good on the outside.

Remember, comparison is the thief of joy. Behind the glamour, or the seemingly flawless lifestyles you see on your Insta squares is a person, just like you. Someone that, at times, will be filled with self-doubt or self-loathing, with despair or confusion. The truth is, it doesn't matter *how* people present themselves, underneath it all, everyone shares profound similarities in their insecurities and fears.

If there's one message we hope you take away from this book, it's this: you're not alone. Yes, you are unique, and only **you** are going through your specific journey. But, ultimately, (as we have all learned since 2020) we are all in this together. Undoubtedly, there is someone else reading this book who, like you, has some work to do to improve their wellbeing, or is looking for some simple tweaks to ensure they stay on top of their game. Either way. This is for you. Let's go!

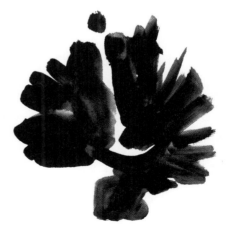

HOW TO BE WELL AUDIT QUESTIONNAIRE

Answer each audit question and mark the column that best fits with your current State of Being. Remember, there are no right or wrong answers, just your truth.

HOW TO WORK OUT YOUR SCORE

Score ZERO for each answer in Column 1

Score 2 for each answer in Column 2

Score 3 for each answer in Column 3

	QUESTION	1	2	3
1	Energy levels?	Low	OK	Great
2	Have you ever been treated for cancer?	Yes – within the past two years	Yes – more than two years ago	No
3	Have you had chemotherapy?	Yes, within the last five years	Yes, more than five years ago	No
4	Are you currently being treated for any chronic medical disease? *	Yes		No
5	Do you have high blood pressure?	Yes	Don't know	No
6	How many alcoholic standard drinks per week do you have?	More than 7	4-7	0-3
7	Has anyone commented that you may drink too much alcohol?	Often	Occasionally	Never
8	Do you smoke?	Yes		No
9	How often do you open your bowels without laxatives?	I'm constipated	Every 2-3 days	Daily
10	Do you buy organic food and personal care products?	No	Occasionally	Over 80% are organic
11	Do you drink 8 glasses of filtered water per day?	No	Occasionally	Always
12	Daily vegetable serves (1 serve equals about ½ cup)	Rarely have them	1-2 serves every day	More than 3 serves daily
13	Do you eat nuts and seeds?	Rarely	A few times per week	Every day
14	Do you have fast food takeaway meals?	Yes. More than 2 times per week	Yes. 1-2 times per week	Rarely. 1-2 times per month

*Chronic diseases include cardiovascular disease, hypertension requiring medication, diabetes, autoimmune disease, any condition requiring regular medical supervision, medication or causing chronic pain.

	QUESTION	1	2	3
15	Do you exercise or do movement that makes you puff?	No	1-2 times per week; more than 4 sessions per week	Up to 4 sessions weekly
16	Do you work regular night shifts?	Yes. More than 5 nights monthly	Yes. Less than 6 nights per month	No
17	How many hours of sleep do you have per night?	6 or less hours	More than 9	7-9 hours
18	Is your body weight a problem? (Brutal honesty here, please)	Too high	Too low	Just right
19	How stressful is life at the moment?	Terrible	OK. Just the usual	Not much stress at all
20	Have you experienced the loss of a significant person (or pet) in the past two years? Or have you experienced a death, divorce or break-up?	Yes		No
21	Do you have someone that you can share your problems and worries with?	No	Maybe	Yes
22	Do you meditate or have other restorative practices in your routine?	Never	Occasionally	Regularly
23	Do you consider your mind to be 'busy'?	All the time	Much of the time	Rarely
24	Do you have a short fuse?	Always	Sometimes	Never
25	Do you find yourself crying or feeling sad for no reason?	Regularly	Occasionally	Rarely
26	Do you put other's needs before your own?	Yes. Always	Yes. Sometimes	Rarely

YOUR HEALTH AUDIT RESULTS

Total up your points for your Health Audit score.

This is your **BASELINE** score. The higher the number, the closer you are to a **Thriving State of Being**. A good way to determine how you are improving in certain areas is to retake this audit every few weeks. A change in your score can be a great incentive to continue on your positive wellness path.

Of course, this table is not a comprehensive assessment of your health and State of Being. We find it very useful to identify the important areas of wellness that require special attention in women's lives. If your score result concerns you, or there are specific areas of your health and wellness you want to work on, please take a look at our Resources (see page 452) to seek out some professional one-on-one guidance.

COME BACK HERE!
You might like to mark this page with a sticky note or bookmark. Then you'll be able to easily refer back here to check your progress against your current State of Being.

SCORE 0 – 35: YOUR CURRENT STATE OF BEING IS DEPLETED

If your score says you are in a **Depleted State of Being**, it's probably no surprise to you. You may even be relieved to finally acknowledge just how run down you have become. Our advice? We prescribe rest, self-care and kindness. However, after months or years of taking care of everyone else and overlooking your own health needs, it may be difficult to know where to start.

As you read on, you'll discover how we can work with you to restore you to optimum health. But firstly, you need to make a commitment to your own health. Which means you will need to prioritise your own self and let go of unhelpful habits that may interfere with the optimal functioning of your body. We hope you are prepared to face some shifts in your perception and in your daily routines. The benefits will be well worth it.

The following chapters will clearly define the **non-negotiable** lifestyle changes that you will need to adopt as part of your recovery to allow your physical body and your emotional self the time and space to heal. While these changes or new practices may feel challenging (or even impossible) at times, please be patient. Trust the process and remind yourself that achieving optimal health may take some time (after all, less than ideal health doesn't tend to happen overnight either).

If you support your body, manage your mind and honestly experience your emotions during this process, your energy will improve and you will be firmly on the healing path. Commit to yourself and become your own best friend. Your goal is to work towards a **Thriving State of Being**. Practice patience until you build momentum. Be brave – your body knows what to do, let it be your guide.

CASE STUDY | DR KAREN

Leanne

State of Being: Depleted

Leanne, a mother of two teenagers, works in her own design business and supports her husband, a self-employed builder. The dominos started to fall after a particularly stressful Easter when her husband broke his leg and was unable to work for several weeks. Leanne entered that winter more run-down than usual. She wasn't sleeping well and found herself waking in the early hours of the morning, her mind already busy with thoughts of her to-do list for the next day. A minor respiratory tract infection came into the household from school, and Leanne had to take to her bed for over a week. She ended up taking a course of antibiotics when the cough extended into its third week.

Several weeks later she made an appointment to see me, worried about some chest pains and shortness of breath. All the standard medical tests, blood pathology and chest X-ray were reported as 'normal'. Instead of reassurance, this lack of explanation for the way she was feeling created a layer of fear, as she struggled to find the energy to care for her family and meet the demands of her business.

Leanne had always been the queen of multitasking, sometimes surviving on only a few hours' sleep a night to meet work deadlines, while caring for her young family. Her frustration at her lack of diagnosis was compounded by poor sleep, despite her ongoing exhaustion. Weeks later she described how even the smallest sound at night could drive her crazy: 'Even my husband's breathing sounds like a freight train in the bedroom at night'. She went on to explain that she had to remove all the clocks in the house because their ticking annoyed her. She found herself on a short fuse with any noise coming from the children as they played their video computer games or watched TV. 'And I can't even remember the smallest things now,' she explained, concerned that there may be a more serious problem with her memory.

On further questioning, Leanne was also frustrated by a new deposit of fat around her middle, even though she had lost her appetite and was eating less. I also noted that her blood pressure was elevated above normal levels for the first time in years.

FROM DEPLETED TO SURVIVING TO THRIVING

So what happened to Leanne? Her road to recovery was a slow and gentle unpacking of her lifestyle habits, to make small ongoing adjustments to her daily routines. These are the strategies we share in this book. Today, Leanne looks back on that time and is grateful that she took the time to prioritise self-care.

WOMEN AND STRESS HORMONES

If you identify with Leanne, take special note of Pillar Three. Then read Chapter 11, **Secret Women's Business – Finding Hormonal Harmony (see page 378)**, which outlines the effect of stress on female hormones and how this may manifest itself. The domino effect of stress on a woman's body and what it does to your female hormones adds a layer of complexity to any health solution. Younger women pay a different price for stress than their older counterparts. But for women of all ages, it can take its toll on your health, happiness, relationships and your ability to get the most out of the day.

SCORE 36 – 60: YOUR CURRENT STATE OF BEING IS SURVIVING

If you score or identify with the **Surviving State of Being**, welcome to the club! There are a lot of members here! And no wonder. Today's world is overwhelming. There can be so many 'to be' and 'to do' lists that life can feel as though you're on a never-ending treadmill. But you can't run forever; your body cannot maintain a stressed survival state permanently. At some point something will give and it's usually your health and your emotional wellbeing.

It's time for you to Be Well: To regain balance in your life, you need to make a commitment to yourself to do everything you can to support your body's natural healing systems. This may require a lifestyle overhaul or simply a shift in perspective. Do you have any habits or ingest any substances that sabotage your body's ability to renew and heal itself? Take a good look at your current 'daily grind'. Your body is likely to be running on stress hormones: this needs to change. The adrenal glands tend to be seriously under the pump for most people in the 'survival' state. This dominos into symptoms that include insomnia and hormonal imbalance – symptoms which are so common in both women and men in the modern world. Much of the content in this book will both assist and challenge you. It could be that your current habit is to adopt the 'I am fine' mantra, but underneath it all you really aren't fine. The consequences simply may not have shown up yet, and you may be heading towards a **Depleted** State of Being.

CASE STUDY | DR KAREN

Lorraine

State of Being: Surviving

Lorraine was always very physically active from a young age. She enjoyed boundless energy and thrived on being busy. In her twenties she was a part-time personal trainer on top of her administration job in the family business. She came to see me for a pre-conception check-up a few months after stopping the contraceptive pill. Her periods were regular but heavier than they had been during the years she'd been on the pill.

During this consultation Lorraine told me about her plans for the future. She intended to fall pregnant in the next six months, work up until two weeks before her due date and would be able to take three months off after having her baby.

I reviewed her daily activity schedule taking notes on some important lifestyle choices that could potentially impact on both optimal health and fertility. Because of her busy lifestyle and long hours at work, followed by her personal training classes, evening meals were often on the run. The meals were usually from convenient takeaway outlets and not particularly nourishing or balanced. Given her long work hours during weekdays, mealtime was often at around 8pm, in front of the television. Her husband kept the same gruelling schedule, and they both would usually fall into bed exhausted at around 10pm, after watching an episode of their favourite Netflix series and checking emails.

Lorraine considered her sleep patterns and quality to be 'good'. She noted that she was so exhausted by bedtime that she was asleep within minutes. Two or three times per week she would wake around 3am with a busy mind, going over the work issues of the previous day and planning her day ahead. The alarm would often wake her just as she was returning to a deep slumber around 5am. She told me that she struggled to get out of bed but felt better after her morning dose of coffee.

When I asked her if she felt stressed, she replied that her busy life energised her. Recently, however, she had noted that her energy levels dipped just after finishing her periods and she felt as though she was on a shorter fuse at work.

LORRAINE'S PATH TO WELLNESS

Whilst Lorraine had a perception that she was healthy – due to being a very fit woman – her sleep patterns, high exercise activities and inconsistent eating habits were leading her down the path of imbalance. This imbalance was affecting her hormonal balance. I counselled her that preconception care was an important component to fertility, a smooth pregnancy and healthy child. We spoke about priorities: the importance of trying to switch some of the more gruelling exercise classes and include some more restorative options; prepare more nourishing meals ahead of time for freezing if she was time-poor; prioritising spending time in her Blue Zone (covered further in Chapter 6, 7 and 8), rather than checking emails before bed and falling asleep watching TV, to decrease her stress levels and offer her a more consistent sleep. I encouraged her to follow the principles we outline for stress resilience in Chapter 8.

Sound familiar? As you read this book you will find more information and helpful advice to help guide you to the path of **Thriving**, the ultimate **State of Being**.

Many women sit in the Surviving State of Being: often unaware of the potential to feel better, and not quite unwell enough to be motivated to actively seek change.

SCORE 61 – 78: YOUR CURRENT STATE OF BEING IS THRIVING

If you score or identify with a **Thriving State of Being**, congratulations! This is a natural State of Being, yet the demands of modern life have made it fragile and rare for many of us to stay here. Strong boundaries and personal commitment are required to maintain this level, and you are clear on what you want and need.

How to continue to Be Well: Even though this is the optimum state we want women to achieve, there's still work to be done to maintain your thriving state. It's important to be vigilant about the messages your body sends you, so pay attention to what it's trying to tell you. Your body is constantly giving you feedback: try to notice anything that feels not quite right. Some messages like changes in the frequency and heaviness of menstrual periods, are impossible to ignore, while others can be quite subtle.

The secret is to 'do a little', before you need to 'do a lot'.

The information in this book will offer insight and strategies to maintain this optimal wellness state. We recommend you familiarise yourself with the other **States of Being** - both **Depleted** and **Surviving** - as it is worthwhile to be aware and mindful of the common saboteurs of wellness.

CASE STUDY | DR KAREN

Nadine

State of Being: Thriving

Nadine, a 34-year-old mother of two, came to see me for a routine check. She was a long-term patient who had breezed through her uncomplicated pregnancies and delivered healthy babies who were now three- and five-years old. She was beginning to wean, but she and her son Oscar were still continuing to enjoy breastfeeds two or three times per week.

Nadine had embraced optimal health choices for most of her adult life. As she was a long-term patient of mine, she understood that her love of hard aerobic exercise was likely to cause stress on her body. She chose to eat organic whole foods, balancing her aerobic exercise with yoga and Pilates classes during the week, whilst being mindful of time management. I also cautioned her that she had youth on her side and that as the years passed, she would need to modify her love of spin classes.

She shared that the main purpose of her visit was to ensure she was in peak condition for an upcoming holiday trek in three months' time. One of the prompts to see me was her mother's recent heart scare.

Nadine seemed an ideal example of a woman in a thriving state. She had great muscle mass and tone and her body weight was perfect for her height. She was sleeping well and felt that her energy levels were good, considering the number of activities she scheduled into her full week.

NADINE'S PATH TO CONTINUED WELLNESS

We did some testing to ensure that Nadine's body could cope with the increased demands required for her very physical holiday. Her results showed good iron stores and healthy levels of key nutrients along with low inflammation markers. Her baseline heart check included an ECG heart tracing and in my opinion she was in good shape for her planned adventure. Nadine was mindful she would need to allow recovery time on her return.

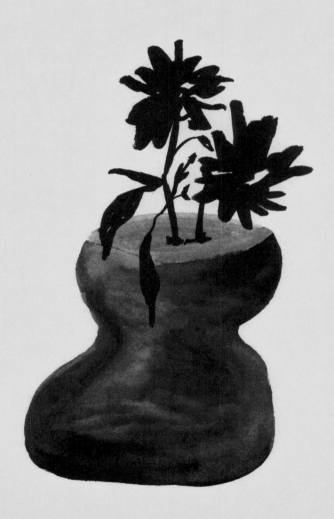

MAINTAINING A THRIVING STATE OF BEING
INVOLVES REGULAR HEALTH AUDITS

Every day you will be confronted with different daily stresses sent to challenge you, as you move through different hormonal phases of your life. While your health goal posts remain the same, your life choices can have subtle impacts on nutrition and hormonal pathways that can sabotage your ability to thrive.

Depleted or Surviving States of Being?
It's time to make some changes.

Now that you have your baseline score, you are ready to move forward through the chapters. Keep a pen and paper handy so that you can take notes of where you need to do the most work and how best to go about it.

Change starts here.

You are entering Pillar One...

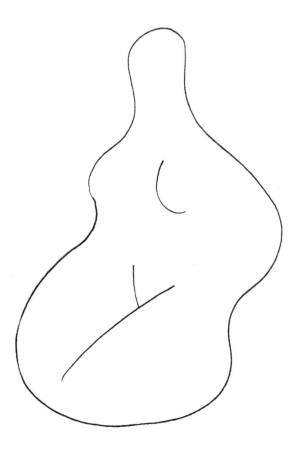

3.
NOURISHMENT

Eat food,
not too much,
mostly plants.

MICHAEL POLLAN

How well do you eat? Do you eat for fuel? For nourishment? For energy? Or do you find emotional comfort in your food? What you eat, how you eat and when you eat are all equally important, and can affect the way your body digests your food, absorbs the ingredients and goodness and, ultimately, how your cells use food to perform their many tasks.

EVERYONE EATS A DIFFERENT MEAL

There is no one-size-fits-all eating plan that will perfectly nourish every single one of us: we are all different, with unique nourishment needs. Heritage, genetics, digestion, stress levels, food allergies and intolerances, metabolic rates and age – all these factors impact the way our bodies process food. It's important to find out what works for you, because your health, wellbeing, mood, energy and self-esteem are directly affected by everything you consume. Both positively and negatively.

There's far more to food than simply energy in versus energy out, and many elements collide to impact your daily intake. Time pressures, level of interest, cooking skills and budget are just some of the things that affect the way you eat. Fad diets, conflicting advice, food habits and beliefs also influence your choices. In fact genetic research shows that those who 'eat right for their genes' are more likely to lead a healthy life, free of chronic disease and that they have less of a battle with body fat. Let's start by investigating if your food intake is fresh and whole, with minimal processing.

THE BUSINESS OF FOOD

Humans have been consuming food for thousands of years. It is only in the last one hundred years of human existence that we have begun to manipulate and change the natural state of our food.

The way in which foods are marketed and advertised has complicated our understanding of them. The more they are processed and the more health claims that are made around what these foods can do, the harder it is to see them for what they really are.

SPOT THE DIFFERENCE

Think of the altered ways an orange and orange juice are presented at the supermarket. The orange will have no packaging and a tag at the front of the shelf stating the price and country of origin. The orange juice will be packaged, with a label stating the brand and promises of vitamins and lack of sugar. Beside the juice will be a range of other juices, with competing claims. Without spending half the day reading nutrition labels, it's hard to know which is the healthiest option.

Of course, the best option is the orange in the fruit and vegetable section, packaged perfectly in its own skin by Mother Nature. In its natural state, the orange provides fibre and other essential elements that help your body absorb the nutrients from the juice without spiking blood sugar levels the way pure juice in a container does.

FOOD: FACTS AND FICTION

Food myths also have a big influence on our perception of foods and why we should be consuming them. Take cow's milk, for example. Many believe that the best way to avoid osteoporosis is by consuming as much cow's milk (and cow's milk products) as possible. For some this is not a problem, but for those with an intolerance this causes more problems than solutions.

Many people have trouble digesting the lactose (sugar) or casein (protein) in cow's milk products. This can be the result of the lack of a gene called the Lactase Persistent Gene or caused by a disruption of the gut lining. This isn't so surprising when you consider that cow's milk is designed to grow calves into very large animals. Although cow's milk is a good source of calcium, it's not the only source. While this mineral plays a role in bone strength, there is more to the osteoporosis story than dairy and calcium alone.

If you have an intolerance to cow's milk, you may find that goats' or sheep milk products do not pose the same health or digestive problems, plus they're a good source of calcium. As goats and sheep are smaller than us, the protein in their milk is easier for us to digest. You should always check with a qualified nutrition expert if you suspect an intolerance or allergy to anything that comes from an udder before you stock the fridge with these alternatives.

HOW NAKED IS YOUR SHOPPING?

To avoid being caught up in the business of food, it's best to consider how far it has progressed from its natural state. The general rule is to choose whole foods which come in the same packaging as created by Mother Nature, and to stay away from human-packaged foods. Don't get sucked into a good marketing campaign by believing the promises on the packaging. Most are, at best, misleading, and some are outrageously untrue. The real truth is that packaged food comes with little to no consideration of nourishment and the finely tuned interplay between your food and your genes. The real food that will nourish your body comes from farms and is found in the fruit and vegetable section, ideally at the farmer's markets or from your own garden. The less your food (and the animals that become food) has been tampered with by humans, the better the food is for you and your family. In an ideal world, pantries should be small and contain only essential items such as whole grains, dried herbs, oils, spices, nuts and seeds. Refrigerators should be large and stacked with clean fresh food.

LEARN TO READ LABELS

Taking control of the foods you buy and consume begins with education. Knowing what to look for on food labels can help you make better, informed choices.

SERVING SIZE

Some food labels swear that their product serving size will suit one person, when in reality it's slightly bigger than that. For instance, a 150g pot of yoghurt is enough for 1½ people. Keep in mind that a serving size is 100g per person (in most instances). By dividing the serving size between one-and-a-bit people, the amount of sugar, fat, salt and calories appears to be lower.

BAKING

Beware of baked goods! If you're buying a product in store, such as chicken that is pre-baked, it may have undergone a cooking process similar to frying. The better option is to bake your ingredients at home where you have greater control over the process.

NO ADDED SUGAR

Possibly the most misleading label of all. The words 'No Added Sugar' doesn't necessarily mean that a product does not contain any sugar. It means that the manufacturer has not added any white sugar or sugar products but sugar can still naturally occur. For example, a two-litre bottle of fruit juice may be labelled with 'no added sugar' but it may contain up to one cup or 250 grams of sugar from the sugar that's already present in fruit.

FAT FREE

Another misleading label. Fat free may mean that sugar and salt have been added to improve the taste. Instead, look for whole fat sources such as olive oil, nuts and seeds.

PRETTY PACKAGING

There's a whole world of science behind the way products are presented to us: any packaging that looks natural, earthy or organic gives buyers the impression that the contents are good for you. And this isn't always the case.

LITE

Leaving aside the dreadful spelling, claims of lite/light doesn't necessarily mean that the product is healthier – it may be that the product is lighter in colour. Instead, look for Mother Nature's products as they have not been processed or altered from their natural state.

KNOW THE ALIASES

Sugar, fat and salt have pseudonyms they act under: fruit juice, milk solids, sodium from garlic are just a few. A rule of thumb: if the words on the label seem overly complicated, then there's probably a better choice available.

FREE-FROM

A product may proclaim that it is sugar-, gluten-, fat-free, natural, organic: and if we're trying to eat healthier we may choose these products, certain that we're making an informed and better purchase. But it's all about the product. For instance, a gluten-free cake is still cake, containing fats, sugars and salt.

NATURAL

When we read this word we logically expect the food would not contain anything that is not good for us. However, this is not the case. There is no regulation around the use of the word 'natural' on food packaging.

FREE RANGE

This term means that the animals are raised in large sheds and have access to the outdoors each day for some unspecified period of time. It could be only for a few minutes and does not assure that the animal ever actually went outdoors to roam freely.

GMO

We strongly recommend that you stay clear of all foods labelled GMO.

Many of the processed foods available in our grocery stores include genetically engineered ingredients.

GMO stands for Genetically Modified Organisms. GMOs have been altered by adding genetic material from different species or making other changes that couldn't happen through traditional breeding. There is no scientific consensus regarding the safety of these foods, despite industry claims.

The weak approval process of new GMO crops in the USA relies solely on testing by the companies. In Australia it is a requirement for foods containing over 1% of GMO of *any* ingredient to be labelled as containing GMO. Foods containing the oils canola or safflower may have traces of genetically modified ingredients. These products are best avoided.

According to the Australian Government Department of Health (at the time of writing) there are currently experimental field plantings of the following foods:

Banana
Barley
Ryegrass
Mustard
Sugar cane
Wheat

In the past there have also been trials of genetically altered rice, clover, maize, poppy, papaya, pineapple and grapevines.

ORGANIC VS NON-ORGANIC

Organic is a prime example of one label that is misused. Mostly, that's because the word 'organic' can mean several different things. It is *not* a guarantee there is an absence of non-organic components within the food. Labels that say certified organic are different. For both food and cosmetics, the 'certified organic' label guarantees the product has been scrutinised vigorously by organic certification third parties.

FOOD HABITS AND BELIEFS

The *way* you ate (not just what you ate) as a child often plays a significant role in establishing your relationship with food as an adult. Parents are teachers, leading both by example and by deciding which foods will be available. From an early age, children learn to manipulate their parents into feeding them food they like to eat, based on taste preferences rather than nutritional value (ice cream, yes! Cabbage, no!). As a child, you may have been rewarded with sugary treats for good behaviour, or to calm you down. Depending on your heritage, your food may have looked different to others and perhaps you were bullied because of the contents of your lunchbox. Such patterns can teach you to have an emotional connection to food.

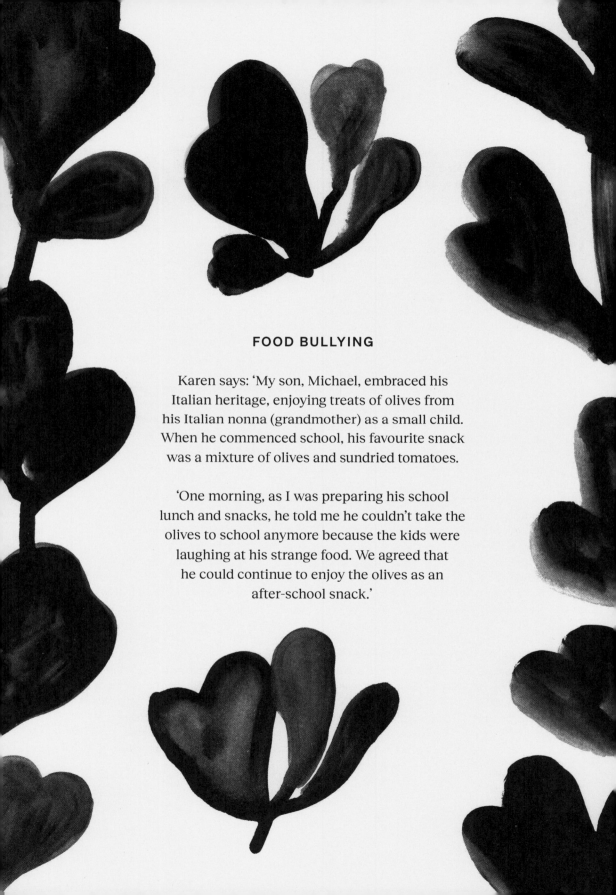

FOOD BULLYING

Karen says: 'My son, Michael, embraced his Italian heritage, enjoying treats of olives from his Italian nonna (grandmother) as a small child. When he commenced school, his favourite snack was a mixture of olives and sundried tomatoes.

'One morning, as I was preparing his school lunch and snacks, he told me he couldn't take the olives to school anymore because the kids were laughing at his strange food. We agreed that he could continue to enjoy the olives as an after-school snack.'

As you grow older, you may have been told to restrict 'naughty or bad' foods to maintain your figure. Welcome food guilt! Add a little peer pressure ordering a burger and fries because that's what everyone else is having, or encouraging others to binge on chocolate with you, and you have a recipe for disaster.

Sadly, the food habits you adopt in your formative years can be hard to shake later in life. One of the common pitfalls seen by dietitians and nutritionists is the indoctrination to 'finish your plate'. This almost certainly had its origins in wartime when food was scarce and more valuable to a family. This food habit gives false messages to your brain about when to stop eating, disconnecting you from your innate sense of fullness.

Not surprisingly, many professionals trained in nutrition say their clients talk more about *why* they eat, rather than *what* they eat. It's the elephant in the room: often the reason people eat (and you may not be aware of this) is emotional. Often there is an unconscious drive. When reaching for a high-fat or sugary snack, do you think: 'I am bored', 'I am stressed', 'I feel unloved', 'I am anxious'?

The prevalence of eating disorders is escalating yearly and they have become major risk factors for lifestyle diseases. These disorders are not always initiated by a hurtful comment around food or body shape. They are very complicated diseases that have some origins in either self-punishment or a desire to control some element of life where there is emotional discomfort or pain. Whether you were overfed and undernourished, or underfed and undernourished, there can be a damaging obsession with food. If you feel that you have a damaged or unhealthy relationship with food, it may help to discuss these issues with your doctor, therapist or ideally a qualified Functional Nutritionist (this is a professional with a tertiary qualification in nutrition or dietetics with a postgraduate wholistic focus on gut health and individual nutritional needs). The difference between a dietitian and a nutritionist is: dietitians are tertiary qualified to diagnose eating disorders and to prescribe diets to treat medical conditions, and are predominately hospital or community based; nutritionists deal with general nutritional advice and can help identify nutritional gaps in your diet and how your body receives and digests your food. Some community-based dietitians also practice as nutritionists.

FAD DIETS

Consumers, especially women, receive so many mixed messages regarding food and the healthiest way to eat: from the media, social media influencers and yes, sometimes by experts in the field. One expert will advise a high-protein diet, another will espouse a low-fat eating plan; one will tell you to consume carbohydrates, while the next will tell you to cut them out. Magazines feature high-sugar, high-fat recipes in one section and then tout the latest diet the 'actor of the moment' follows in another. No wonder everyone is confused!

The diet industry is worth USD 288.25 billion worldwide.

Know this. Fad diets are a multi-billion-dollar industry. Keep tabs on them long enough and you'll begin to notice that diet crazes are recycled every few years with a slight twist and marketed under a different name. The next generation takes the bait and bends to the pressure of the 'body perfect' message, keeping the cycle going. Meanwhile, obesity and diabetes rates rise alarmingly, causing major health complications.

Getting off this dieting cycle involves little more than common sense, awareness and commitment.

5 WAYS
TO GET OFF
THE FAD DIETING
MERRY-GO-ROUND

1.
Stop listening to external voices

The only advice you should follow is from a health professional. Block influencers or information on social media that promises a 'quick fix' or is spruiking the latest health fad.

2.
Start listening to your internal voice

Your body will tell you what it needs. Listen to it. Your body is the best barometer and communicator for which foods we cannot digest well or tolerate. One way to do this is by keeping a food and mood diary, noting what you've eaten and how you feel physically and emotionally afterwards. This can help you determine if a pattern emerges.

3.
Only take advice from nutritionally qualified experts

A qualified Functional Nutritionist or naturopath is your best source for advice and diagnosis surrounding issues such as how to reduce your body fat levels, improve your sleep, increase muscle mass as well as on food intolerances or sensitivities.

Beware! A nutritionist who has done a 12-month course (perhaps online) will not be as informed as a nutritionist who has a university degree. And it is best to ensure that a qualified dietitian is well versed in all aspects of nutritional science. Some practitioners trained in this field show little to no preference for the quality of food you eat; they are more concerned with a 'calories in, calories out' approach, which is not necessarily the best blanket advice.

It is always best to source professional and qualified advice through someone who has a holistic approach to nutritional science. Look for a dietitian with a postgraduate study in clinical nutrition. Or ideally a dietitian, nutritionist or naturopath who is trained in Nutrigenomics (the science of how your food talks to your genes, see Chapter 12 for further information). As research and discoveries in medical science continue to develop, valid nutritional advice must consider your unique genetic landscape and gut microbiome.

4.
Question your beliefs

Just because you have always eaten a certain way doesn't mean that your eating habits couldn't benefit from a makeover. Take note and be mindful of how you think about certain foods. Is there a memory associated with a particular food or ingredient: a reward, a punishment or a cultural preference?

While it is glorious to retain your heritage and eat foods that represent either tradition or are steeped in meaning, you may sometimes be guilted into eating them by well-meaning loved ones. In many cultures, there is a belief connecting the ritual of food preparation and sharing of food with the giving of love. This can be very tricky to navigate; many traditional foods are overly nutrient-dense and were used historically to provide sustenance for heavy physical work outdoors in cooler climates. Of course, embrace the ritual of food with family and community, just remember to balance your food intake on either side of the celebration. It is what you do most of the time that will impact your body over time.

5.
Purchase, prepare and prioritise

There are three main factors that affect your health: stress, daily movement, and what and how much you eat. Without nutrients, your body can't repair itself and give you energy. Your body needs protein, carbohydrates, whole fats, vitamins, minerals, prebiotics, probiotics and fibre (and that's just for starters!) every day to maintain all its functions. All fad diets fail to provide essential trace minerals and vitamins by encouraging you to cut out one or more of these food groups. Avoiding certain food groups long term should always be under the advice of a qualified nutritional professional. Remember: your body is a biological living organism that knows what to do every minute of every day. It has its own innate wisdom - all you have to do is feed it real food.

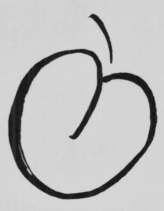

RESTRICTIVE DIETS: WHAT'S MISSING FROM YOUR DAILY INTAKE?

DIET	DESCRIPTION	DEFICIENCY
PALEO	No grains, no legumes, high protein, whole fats, low carb	Calcium Magnesium Folate Iron Iodine
ATKINS	High saturated fat, high protein, low carb	Fibre B-vitamins – thiamine and folate Vitamin C Iron Magnesium
KETO	High fat, low carb	Vitamins A, C and B-vitamins – thiamine and folate Fibre
FODMAP	Excludes fructose and small sugars	Antioxidants Prebiotic sugars that feed your microbiome (good gut bacteria) – this can domino into long-term changes in gut microbiome balance.
GAPS	Excludes grains, starchy vegetables and dairy	Fibre Calcium

DIET	DESCRIPTION	DEFICIENCY
VEGAN	Excludes all animal products	Vitamin B12 Iron Protein Vitamin D Omega 3 fatty acids Iodine Calcium Zinc
VEGETARIAN	Excludes all animal products except eggs and dairy	Vitamin B12 Calcium Iron Zinc Vitamin D Omega 3 fatty acids Protein
DASH	Dietary Approaches to Stop Hypertension – Low sodium diet – salt restriction	Low sodium can be a problem for some people on medication that also lowers blood sodium levels. Overall, an acceptable approach to reducing the risk of hypertension
ORNISH	Excludes all fats and oils, nuts, seeds, meat, fish and poultry – used to reduce cholesterol	Vitamin E Calcium Zinc Vitamin B12 Omega 3 fatty acids

A diet without all the nutrients is like baking without all the ingredients. You can still make a cake, but it will not be the best possible cake. It will merely be a lesser version of the original recipe.

HOW TO EAT REAL

There is a real cost when we do not prioritise the quality and balance of our food: it's called lifestyle disease. Your health and your family's health – not to mention the effect your shopping dollar can have on a local supplier – is dependent on what is in the fridge and in the pantry.

- Buy certified organic as much as possible
- Buy local
- Eat seasonally
- Buy from farmers who raise their animals and kill them ethically
- Buy products that aren't over-packaged (and take your own bags whenever shopping)

A WORD ON VEGAN AND VEGETARIAN DIETS

Lifestyle choices need to fit into your values and how you choose to live in the world. For sustainability and humane reasons, many people choose to exclude any form of animal protein from their diets. We acknowledge and support the passion and commitment these diets take, yet have met many who have not got the nutritional balance right. Following this diet while still getting all the nutrients your body needs can be a complicated art form.

If you are considering a vegan or vegetarian lifestyle, or if you already follow this diet, we strongly encourage you to get some practical advice from a qualified nutritionist to ensure you receive all the essential nutrients you need, either by clever food combining or supplementation if required.

Choose whole fresh foods and be creative. Include a variety of different plant protein sources as nutritional balance is especially important for you to thrive. Avoid the heavily processed plant-based options and meat alternatives that are gaining popularity and becoming more readily available. We cannot trust that food manufacturers have nutrition as a priority when they are delivering new products to capture a market, so it is best to stick to whole foods in their natural form.

THE SUGAR FIX

Is there any time you should or could eat sugar? Or are foods containing sugar forever banned from our shopping lists? We asked **Carolina Rossi**, Holistic Dietitian and Functional Nutritionist, to explain:

'Many of my clients say they're confused about sugar and its role in our body. Add sweeteners into the mix, and the confusion is understandable. Firstly, what is sugar? It's a carbohydrate, and carbohydrates are your body's first source of energy, essential for the optimal function of your brain, kidneys and red blood cells. If your diet is too restricted in carbohydrates, you compromise your body's ability to supply glucose to these organs and cells. It is forced to use another method of making glucose, called gluconeogenesis, which involves converting amino acids (the building blocks of protein) into glucose. This is not ideal, because the waste products of gluconeogenesis put pressure on your organs of elimination. Note: you really want to "save" your amino acids to build hormones, enzymes and muscles.'

HOW INSULIN WORKS

The carbohydrate food family releases glucose into our bloodstream. Blood glucose levels increase from the normal baseline.

Rising blood glucose signals the pancreas to produce insulin. Insulin acts as a key to unlock body cells and let in glucose.

Glucose leaves the bloodstream and enters cells. Blood glucose levels reduce to baseline.

Cells turn glucose into energy.

Simple sugars, such as white sugar and those found in white bread, pasta, chocolate, sweets and other processed foods, can lead to too much glucose in the body. This is because these simple sugars are absorbed quickly across even the unhealthiest bowel wall. When this happens, a fat-storage hormone called insulin is produced. Insulin's role is to facilitate the movement of sugar into the cell, which is then to be used to produce energy. If the blood is hit with a large delivery of dietary sugar, your insulin will surge in response. This can create a domino effect on health where the insulin can overshoot the mark and force blood glucose levels to fall too far.

This state of low blood sugar is called hypoglycaemia and can create the following symptoms:

- Light-headedness
- Feeling of overwhelming dread (pushes the stress response)
- Nausea and vomiting
- Profuse sweating
- Inability to concentrate or stay on task

IS THERE SUCH A THING AS GOOD SUGARS?

Sugars that are found in whole foods, such as sweet potatoes, brown rice, spelt and beetroot, require less insulin to process. Because they also contain fibre, the sugars are released more slowly into your bloodstream. So you'll have less 'spikes' of energy, followed by a slump. Whole foods (those foods that are in their natural state) also contain important minerals and vitamins, such as B vitamins, which improve the efficiency of sugar metabolism.

SMART SUGAR SWAPS
THE BEST SOURCES OF CARBOHYDRATES FOR YOU

SWAP	HEALTHIER CHOICE
Pasta	Brown, black or wild rice, quinoa
Dried fruit	Fresh, organic fruit and berries
Potatoes	Sweet potato, legumes
Cow's milk, yoghurt, cheese	Sheep and goat yoghurt, cheese

The secret to weight gain and loss, and the ability to maintain an ideal body fat percentage is to keep insulin under control.

ARTIFICIAL SWEETENERS – YAY OR NAY?

Artificial sweeteners are chemicals that are best avoided as they increase the toxic load in your body. They're also particularly high liver loaders, so your body takes a long time to process and eliminate them. Most artificial sweeteners contain aspartame, which is broken down into formaldehyde, a chemical that can be toxic to the brain when mixed with common food colourings. Studies have shown that aspartame impairs memory and increases oxidative stress in the brain. The impaired memory performance is associated with reducing the brain's access to its much-needed fuel, glucose. It also worsens insulin sensitivity and has been linked to diabetes and weight gain.

WHY YOU SHOULD BIN THESE SUGAR ALTERNATIVES

SUCRALOSE (FOUND IN SOME ARTIFICIAL SWEETENERS)	Produced by chlorinating sucrose (ordinary table sugar).	Can impair liver detoxification pathways.
XYLITOL, SORBITOL AND ERYTHRITOL	A result of the alcohols made through the fermentation process of plant materials.	Can cause gastrointestinal distress, including profuse diarrhoea.
HIGH-FRUCTOSE CORN SUGAR	Artificial sugar made from corn syrup.	Is stored as fat in your liver, compromising detoxification and functionality. It also leads to leptin resistance (the hormone that regulates your appetite). Linked to Metabolic Syndrome and increased risk of heart disease.

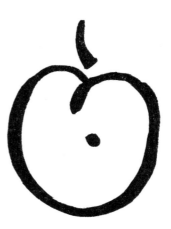

EXPLORE THE TASTY WORLD OF NATURAL SWEETENERS

Swap sugar for a natural alternative that still brings some sweetness to the table without any of the hidden health hazards.

RAW HONEY

A combination of fructose and glucose. It has higher fructose levels than maple syrup, but it contains antioxidants and other protective properties (it is antibacterial and alleviates allergies). Always choose raw honey for its higher nutrient and antioxidant content.

MAPLE SYRUP

High in nutrients and antioxidants. Contains anti-inflammatory properties and may help regulate blood sugar. Check the label for 'pure maple syrup', rather than the imitation maple-flavoured syrup.

STEVIA

A good alternative for diabetics. Stevia is derived from a plant and has been used as a sweetener for hundreds of years. Available in tablets or liquid, it has no calories and is 200 times sweeter than sugar in the same concentration. Check the label to ensure you're buying 100 per cent stevia.

(Note that large amounts of Stevia is not recommended, especially for pregnant women.)

MONK FRUIT

This natural sweetener is derived from its namesake fruit. It is a good substitute for sugar, especially for those needing to avoid all sugars. It does not activate the insulin pathways and the aftertaste is not as bitter as Stevia.

Honey and maple syrup may be better alternatives to sugar but they are still energy dense and should be used sparingly.

RETRAINING YOUR BRAIN

Why is sugar so damn addictive? Sugar is, for many, the demon of the pantry. It calls us at strange times of day and night, when we're stressed, tired, hormonal, bored or anxious. Unfortunately, there's no way to hide from the truth. Sugar is bad for you, despite how good it feels eating it. When you consume sugar, the dopamine receptors (the part of your brain that dictates desire and addiction) are activated. **This is the very same area of the brain that lights up in people who have an addiction to drugs such as cocaine, heroin and nicotine.**

The pleasure point of the brain lies deep within the ancient section of your brain responsible for the control of bodily functions and hormones. This is the amygdala, the emotional sensor and centre for sexual pleasure, cravings, reward and focus. This is also the home of dopamine, one of our many powerful neuroactive, feel-good hormones. Just like cocaine, codeine, caffeine, alcohol, nicotine and heroin, sugar stimulates the dopamine receptors in our brain. This is the part that perceives rewards and enables cravings.

Alongside coffee, sugar is probably the most universally available and socially acceptable dopamine stimulator.

Here's how the addictive cycle works. The constant bombardment by sugar of the receptor site for dopamine over time results in a depletion of the dopamine stores. The ONLY way to feel that good again is to continually batter the cells in the midbrain with more sugar. This goes way beyond what we need for nourishment or to satisfy hunger.

Sugar is one of the most significant saboteurs of wellness.

It's not always been this way. Our relationship with food has changed immeasurably during the past 30 years. Even though we can get Netflix on demand, our bodies are still chemically primitive.

WHAT SUGAR DOES TO YOUR BODY

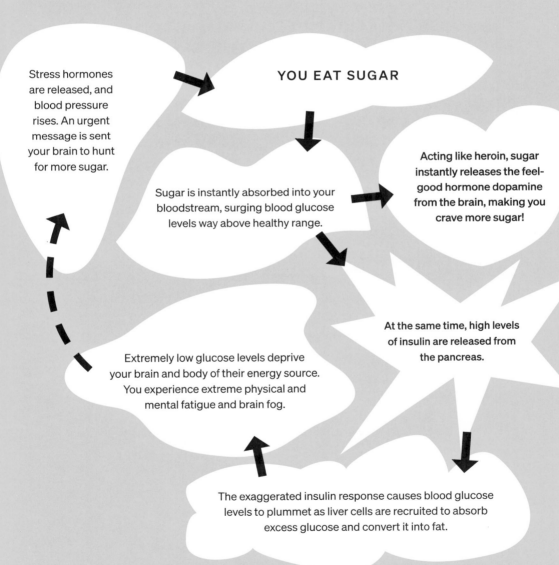

Stress hormones are released, and blood pressure rises. An urgent message is sent your brain to hunt for more sugar.

YOU EAT SUGAR

Sugar is instantly absorbed into your bloodstream, surging blood glucose levels way above healthy range.

Acting like heroin, sugar instantly releases the feel-good hormone dopamine from the brain, making you crave more sugar!

At the same time, high levels of insulin are released from the pancreas.

Extremely low glucose levels deprive your brain and body of their energy source. You experience extreme physical and mental fatigue and brain fog.

The exaggerated insulin response causes blood glucose levels to plummet as liver cells are recruited to absorb excess glucose and convert it into fat.

FIRST, A BRIEF HISTORY LESSON

The most significant change in our dietary choices over the past 30 years has been our increased love of refined sugar found in processed foods and carbonated soft drinks. Simple table sugar is sucrose and is broken down in the body to become glucose and fructose.

THE FACTS ON FRUCTOSE

Fructose is cheap and mooted as a 'natural sugar' by the food industry, but this demon is far from sweet. Unlike glucose, fructose relies solely on the liver to metabolise it, making it **as potent as alcohol** in its demands on the liver. This can have a domino effect on the delicate balance of hormonal plays and toxin degradation as the liver has to choose between two jobs: that of hormonal balance, or the processing and elimination of toxic by-products of fructose.

We are facing a health nightmare with the emergence of the following links between ill-health and fructose:

- A connection to increased cancer cell metabolism
- Links to diabetes, obesity and heart disease
- Hypertension in children

FRUIT AND FRUCTOSE

Most fruit provides fructose as the end point. However fruit should never be excluded from a healthy diet, unless instructed by a qualified nutritionist or dietitian. Fruit also contains varying amounts of glucose as well as a large variety of vitamins and minerals essential for optimal health. The balance of both fructose and glucose in fruits aids the healthy metabolism of fruit fructose.

FODMAP DIETS – (THIS STANDS FOR FERMENTABLE OLIGOSACCHARIDES, DISACCHARIDES, MONOSACCHARIDES AND POLYOLS)

A FODMAP diet is a medically prescribed diet that excludes certain high-fructose fruits and vegetables. FODMAP is not a 'forever' diet and was never designed to be one. Resting the gut from fructose allows healing of the gut wall and eventually the re-introduction of this important food family. Following a FODMAP diet for longer than a few months excludes vital anti-oxidants, fibre, nutrients and prebiotics (food for your microbiome). In other words, FODMAP is not a healthy diet long-term.

HIGH-FRUCTOSE CORN SYRUP

If you've been reading your food labels you may have noticed the words 'high-fructose corn syrup' which is becoming increasingly present in processed foods. The presence of this ingredient has been linked with gut symptoms that mimic irritable bowel syndrome and, more worryingly, fatty liver disease. Avoid foods containing this ingredient as much as you possibly can.

SUGAR OR SHOES – YOU CHOOSE

This is probably a good time to talk about retail therapy. Interestingly, shoe shopping seems to be the proven therapy that most tickles our dopamine receptors in a similar way to sugar. Not that we're advocating swapping one addiction for another. Just saying...

SWEET AND LOW

Are you addicted to sugar? Take our quick test to find out if you have an unhealthy reliance on the white stuff.

Do you:

Feel the need to eat every few hours?

Find that you're unable to concentrate mid-morning?

Need a sugary snack for extra energy around 3pm?

Get 'hangry' between meals or around 5pm?

Feel shaky or dizzy if you haven't eaten
for a couple of hours?

Feel energised, or conversely exhausted, after a meal?

Rely on caffeine or sugar to power you through your day?

If you've answered 'Yes' to two or more of these, we suggest you look at detoxifying your diet to eliminate sugar. A clear-out of sugary snacks from your cupboard is your first step to a cleaner, healthier you. It's natural to want sugar – even our ancestors craved a sweet hit (albeit from fruit rather than a packaged chocolate bar).

A NOTE ON DETOX (WITHDRAWAL) FROM SUGAR

Although Type 2 diabetes and sugar addiction are completely different beasts, the end game is the same: we want smooth blood sugar levels throughout the waking day, good nutrient levels and food choices, reduced stress and balanced movement. For those who have the Type 2 diabetic genes loaded into their family tree, faulty sugar processing pathways will be one of the environmental triggers for the onset of diabetes. It's not surprising that the solutions for sugar addiction follow the same guidelines to both prevent the disease and improve the health of Type 2 diabetics.

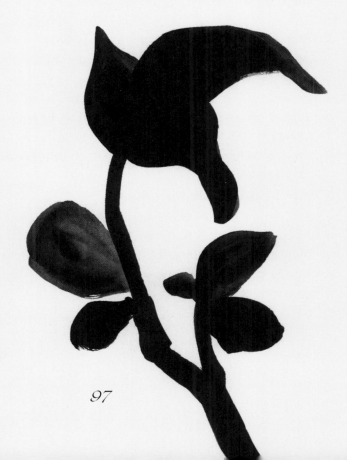

STAY SWEET

6 EASY CHANGES TO CANCEL YOUR SUGAR ADDICTION

1   Adopt a plant-based diet.

2   Limit your daily fructose intake to less than 15g. This allows for up to three serves of fruit per day. Remember, one serve is a piece of fruit.

3   Stop all processed forms of sugars. Avoid glucose, fructose in liquid or powdered form, as well as white or raw sugar. Check your labels!

4   Replace sugar with a natural sweetener such as Stevia or monk fruit. This can help if you can't go cold turkey. Keep Stevia to less than three serves per day and use liquid Stevia in preference to tablets. Highly processed Stevia has been linked to chronic headaches.

5   Never grocery shop when hungry.

6   Keep a nut trail mix handy for those low blood sugar moments - it'll help stop you reaching for the chocolate, candies or biscuits. Make sure it is 90 per cent nuts and seeds with no more than 10 per cent chopped dried fruits.

KEEPING THE KIDS SWEET

Children learn from the lifestyle they're raised in. If they grow up snacking on potato crisps and drinking lemonade, this will be their norm. If there is only nourishing food in the fridge and pantry, however, they *will* eat it if they're hungry (apart from a few stubborn exceptions). If there is no soft drink, juice or cordial, they *will* drink water when they're thirsty. This may mean that we, as adults, need to change our own often fiercely protected, less-than-ideal food habits. Saying it's okay for you (or other members of your family) to eat chocolate biscuits for afternoon tea – when they're not allowed – sends a confusing message to them.

AGREE ON A FAMILY MENU

Which foods would you like your family to eat on a regular basis (from main meals to snacks)? Creating some food guidelines and a healthy framework can help when you are shopping or planning meals. Look at food swaps for healthier substitutes – it's not about deprivation and a tasteless diet.

AGREE ON A 'FOOD LANGUAGE' WITH YOUR FAMILY

Discuss the way you will talk about food on an educational and emotional level as well. For instance, try to avoid using terms such as 'it will make you fat' or 'you will get fat if you eat that'. A positive approach that involves messages such as: 'Yes, that is delicious, but it's a "sometimes food" because it does not help your body grow and be healthy' is far more constructive. Using terminology like 'sometimes food' and 'everyday food' helps to teach healthy food habits without the negative messages that are associated with good and bad behaviour and guilt.

CASE STUDY | SHARON

GIVE KIDS
A HEALTHY START

I remember hearing my 11-year-old daughter tell a friend who was staying over for the night that there was no food in our house. In fact, the pantry and fridge were full of food, but none of it was packaged, convenience food. There were always nuts, seeds, fruit, cheese, chopped celery and carrot, hummus, dates, dried apricots, homemade peanut butter, yoghurt and coconut to snack on. There was plenty to eat if she was hungry, yet as an impressionable child she wanted the cleverly marketed, neatly packaged, processed foods that were full of sugar and salt, offering little nourishment. I did buy such items occasionally, but they were not in the shopping trolley every week. Sure, we argued about it at times and I know she felt like she was missing out, but now, as a healthy adult, she thanks for me for having the courage to stick it out and has now embarked on this journey with her own child.

The five Eat for Life principles

In order to 'Eat for Life' we need to return to the way humans have typically eaten throughout history. Even if you don't read any further than these points, try to remember these simple pieces of advice:

1   Eat mostly **plants**.

2   **Include** some protein in each meal.

3   **Whole fats** are good for you. They're found in avocado, olive oil, nuts and seeds.

4   **Carbohydrates** are not the devil. You need them for good brain function and myriad other body processes.

5   **Stop** eating convenient, packaged and processed foods.

The following guidelines will help you incorporate the Eat for Life principles.

GUIDELINE A: EAT FOOD IN ITS NATURAL STATE

GUIDELINE B: EAT CONSISTENTLY EVERY DAY

GUIDELINE C: EAT PROTEIN, FATS AND CARBOHYDRATES AT EVERY MEAL

GUIDELINE D: EAT SLOWLY AND NOT TOO MUCH AT EACH MEAL

GUIDELINE E: FOLLOW THE S.L.O.W FOOD PRINCIPLE

GUIDELINE F: ENJOY THE FREEDOM OF OUR 80:20 RULE

Let's drill down into the details of these guidelines.

GUIDELINE A

Eat foods that are still in their natural state, as Mother Nature intended.

Make food a priority. Cook and eat together if you live with others or make the effort to cook nourishing meals for yourself.

Remember **food is nourishment**. Look at it as your friend, rather than foe. It's not something to be avoided for weight loss, but better choices will improve your health and overall wellbeing.

Spend time at local farmer's markets to find fresh produce in its natural state. Your trolley in the supermarket should be filled with fresh produce. Avoid the temptation of the aisles containing processed and packaged food. Review our suggestions on page 73 and take pride in filling your refrigerator with naked food.

GUIDELINE B

Eat consistently every single day.

Setting up a positive routine with your mealtimes (no skipping breakfast or lunch!) is imperative for wellbeing. Follow our tips for each meal on the following pages.

Breakfast

Breakfast literally means 'break your fast', used historically to define the first meal of the day. This means there is no set time to eat breakfast, although farmers and athletes tend to eat early for sustenance. Those with the right genome (see chapter 12 for more information on gene testing) do well with intermittent fasting, so breakfast can be pushed out to mid-morning. Interestingly, a well-known breakfast cereal manufacturer coined the phrase 'breakfast is the most important meal of the day' which became the standard thinking around breakfast. So yes it is important to 'break your fast' – just choose a time that suits your metabolism.

YOUR BEST BREAKFAST CHOICES:

- Avoid packaged and processed breakfast cereals. Choose good-quality whole grains such as non-sweetened muesli, raw oats or seeds such as quinoa, and nuts with minimal or ideally no dried fruit.
- One serving of fruit is sufficient.
- Eat the whole egg. Mother Nature packaged this food perfectly.
- Avoid disguised sugar, such as jam and tomato sauce.
- Include some green leafy vegetables and/or herbs.
- One piece of good-quality toast or bread is sufficient. Avoid highly processed breads. Instead, look for wholegrain bread, ideally gluten-free or naturally fermented sourdough. Or, switch out the bread and choose some starchy vegetables, brown rice or legumes instead.
- Protein should come from natural sources such as meat, chicken, nut milks, rice, eggs and fish rather than processed protein powders.
- Coffee and tea are best consumed 20 minutes before or after the meal, not while you're eating, as this improves the digestion of the food you consume.
- A smoothie or homemade vegetable juice is a convenience option for the odd occasion. Liquid meals do not fire up the digestive process or increase metabolism.
- Avoid commercially packaged fruit juices. These simple sugars enter the bloodstream too fast and drive up glucose levels stimulating insulin pathways, driving inflammation and adding extra calories with little nutritional value.

Lunch

- Your lunch should look similar in size and have the same balance as your dinner. Do not fall into the trap of skipping lunch or treating it as a snack, as this will usually lead to overeating at dinner, or snacking before or after dinner.

- Avoid eating at your desk or while you are working or doing a task. Taking time out from work and tasks to fuel your body is an essential part of maintaining your productivity and managing pressure.

- Prepare your work lunch the night before or earlier that morning rather than ordering take-away foods. If you are time-poor, prepare additional protein and starchy carbohydrates at dinner, put them in airtight glass containers and add some salad/vegetable options. In winter, leftover soup or casserole is perfect for lunch the next day.

- If you have to buy your lunch, avoid too much bread, white rice and/or fried foods. Fried foods can drive inflammatory pathways in cells for up to 48 hours after the meal. Inflammation in the body increases the risk of chronic disease and is something we want to reduce. Good choices are grains like brown rice, a selection of vegetables (include starchy veggies, such as sweet potato), or add legumes like beans if there is no form of grain, some protein and green leafy vegetables. If soup is an option, choose a chunky, hearty one that requires you to chew.

- This may not work for everyone, but you could ask if your workplace will provide a slow-cooker in the kitchen. You can set up a roster with interested colleagues, and take turns bringing in pre-prepared ingredients and loading it up in the morning. It will cook while you work and be ready for lunch. This is an excellent option for winter.

Dinner

- Your evening meal should be eaten at the table, away from the television, computer and phone.

- Eat as a family whenever you can – sharing food is a wonderful way to connect with each other. Eating together has always been a ritual and family tradition even in ancient times.

- Choose a balanced meal (a protein and three vegetables), using a wide variety of ingredients to ensure you're getting a mix of nutrients. Enjoy mainly leafy green veg and herbs, and opt for fish or chicken over red meat, which is best kept to one or two meals per week. Try stir-fries served with brown rice, or fish or chicken served with a side of steamed vegetables and a whole baked potato.

- Choose seasonal vegetables and mix them up as often as you can. Include lots of different-coloured vegetables to ensure you receive a variety of vitamins and minerals from your meals.

- Vegans and vegetarians: include a nut, grain, legume and seed to receive all the essential amino acids you need from these plant-based proteins.

- Try to avoid snacks and dessert after dinner. If you do crave something sweet, try baking a whole apple with a sprinkle of cinnamon.

DEVICES AND YOUR DIET

We eat 30 to 60 per cent more when eating in front of the TV or a device.

Ban technology at mealtimes to bring focus to eating and chewing food. Making sure you're masticating your food properly is the cornerstone to improving digestion, helping to heal gut issues and, most importantly, feeding the gut microbiome. Sit down with your family to enjoy a meal and share stories about the day.

SMART SNACKS

What you eat between meals (if you eat at all) may be your biggest downfall. Often we reach for sugary, calorie- and fat-laden snacks to fuel us. Functional Nutritionist Carolina Rossi shares some healthy but filling snack ideas.

- Don't justify eating less at lunch so you can have cake at afternoon tea. This isn't balanced eating, it's emotive.

- Most packaged snacks will affect your blood sugar levels, mood and energy. Avoid!

IDEAS FOR BETTER SNACKS

- One serving of fruit
- Handful of nuts (if you've been very active, have both a piece of fruit *and* nuts)
- 1 cup (250ml) organic vegetable juice or vegetable-based smoothie. Add a small handful of nuts to slow down the absorption of sugar from the gut
- Hummus with vegetable sticks (carrots and celery)
- ¼ avocado and tomato on wholegrain crackers
- Hard-boiled egg

GUIDELINE C

Repeat after us:
protein, fat and carbohydrates

Every meal and snack you enjoy should contain some protein, fat and carbohydrate.

PROTEIN

Protein is anything that has flown, walked or swum, although legumes and grains can be good sources, too.

WHICH PROTEIN IS BEST FOR YOU:
Choose protein sources based on your ability to digest and eliminate them effectively (see You and Your Gut, page 125). Vegans, vegetarians, veg-aquarians or anybody who avoids certain proteins, should include legumes, nuts, seeds and grains with each meal.

WHAT TO AVOID:
Protein powders are processed foods that may contain additives such as sugar or artificial ingredients. They are not a good substitute for real whole foods, and are a fad that should be avoided - you can get all the protein you need from natural sources.

FAT

Whole fats are either saturated, monounsaturated and polyunsaturated, and each one of these has subcategories.

WHICH FAT IS BEST FOR YOU:
You need a balanced combination of whole fats to support your immune system, as fats protect against inflammation. Fats also provide a coating around every cell in our body. All the experts we know agree that 'fat does not make you fat'.

- **Essential fats** are whole fats such as nuts, seeds, avocado, egg yolk, organic oils, tahini and butter.

- **Good fats** are also found in organic grass-fed red meat and chicken, fish and seafood from clean waters.

Thirty per cent of your daily food intake should come from whole fats. These include (ideally certified organic) nuts, seeds, avocado, olive oil, butter, tahini and coconut. Whole fat is also found in meats, fish and chicken.

THE F-WORD

Not all fats are good. Avoid any food that has been deep-fried or cooked in oil at a high heat that has shown signs of smoking during cooking. The high heating process produces destructive trans-fats and hydrogenated fats. These denatured fats are also found in abundance in packaged, fast and takeaway foods (think potato crisps... sorry). These guys are the big baddies; they will literally make you sick because they drive up inflammation in your body for up to 48 hours. Inflammation is the breeding ground for all chronic diseases.

SHOULD I BE EATING ANIMAL PROTEIN?

If you do eat meat and chicken, we suggest buying grass-fed, free range and ideally organically raised. Like humans, animals are at their healthiest when they are in their natural environment munching on what Mother Nature intended them to eat. Imagine a cow eating grass in a large paddock where it roams with a herd and lives in the sunshine and rain – this is how cows are designed to live, with minimal stress.

Animals, birds and fish that are caged, overfed with grain or alternative foods, are often fatter and more stressed. A stressed animal will have a compromised immune system and is more vulnerable to infections and illness. This means they may require antibiotics. These can still be present in the animals on slaughter unless the farmer practices a purging process in the days prior to slaughter. Often these pharmaceuticals are still present in that animal's fat cells.

Treated animals, including birds and fish, have also been exposed to various pesticides and chemicals. Like humans, these toxins are stored in the fat cells in their body to protect their organs from toxic exposure. Avoid grain-fed meats and consider how and where the animal or bird has been raised before you eat the fat.

INFLAMMATION AND YOUR DIET

Avoid all margarines, including those that claim health benefits. In 2013 a major study involving 458 men in Sydney, Australia was cut short when the treated group began showing an increase in death rates and cardiovascular events such as heart attacks and stroke. This randomised controlled trial called the Sydney Diet Heart Study replaced butter with polyunsaturated margarine derived from safflower. The results proved that the recommendations to stop eating butter, a saturated fat, and substitute with polyunsaturated margarine was the wrong advice.

In 2016, research scientist CE Ramsden revisited unpublished data on polyunsaturated fats and heart disease and came to the same conclusion as the Sydney Diet Heart Study. This led to experts recommending a complete revision of current heart health recommendations about margarines. Sadly, more than five years after the original Sydney Diet Heart Study, the myths about margarine being a healthy spread option continue.

Margarines that claim to lower cholesterol are actually basing their claims on solid research. These products do lower cholesterol, but they do not reduce the risk of heart attack and stroke. In fact, revised data in another heart study, the Minnesota Coronary Experiment, found that as cholesterol levels fell in the group consuming the margarine, the death rate from heart attacks went up, not down. It seems the altered fats in margarine are the type of fats that increase inflammation, particularly in the coronary arteries. This is another example of clever marketing allowing the consumer to make the giant leap to presumed health benefits that don't exist. Even worse, these products aggravate the very disease they were supposed to prevent.

How do you navigate this paradox?
Follow the evidence:

- Saturated fats like butter can be part of a healthy diet and need to be capped at 30 per cent of your daily fat intake.
- Increasing extra-virgin organic olive oil, avocados, nuts and seeds has been proven to reduce cardiovascular risk.
- Avoid margarines as they have been shown in research to increase cardiovascular risk, even when they result in a lowered cholesterol score in lab testing.

WHAT ABOUT WAGYU?

A cow that has been physically contained and overfed with grain to achieve the marbling affect in the meat is a very unhealthy obese cow and probably stressed by its environment. This meat may be extremely tasty but, from a nutritional perspective, this meat is in no way as healthy as grass-fed organically raised meat.

CARBOHYDRATES

Carbohydrates grow. That's a very simple way to understand what carbohydrates are: plants, pulses, grains, some seeds, vegetables, herbs and fruits all fall into this category. Some carbohydrates have a higher energy density (calories per bite) than others, such as starchy vegetables like corn, peas, potato and grain. Other carbohydrates are mostly water and have a lower energy density, such as green leafy vegetables and herbs. It's important to eat a mixture of the two for a balanced diet.

You've probably been led to believe that all carbohydrates are bad. However, we need to have a certain amount of carbohydrates in a balanced diet to receive all our micronutrients (vitamins and minerals). The best way to consider your carb intake? Eat a rainbow of food, and you'll have your micronutrients covered.

But what about other carbs, we hear you cry? Include just one starchy carb with each meal or have a small amount of two. (Two servings may be more appropriate if you have a fast metabolism, do hard manual labour or have a high exercise output.) For example, if you are having sweet potato for lunch or dinner, avoid corn or just have a small amount of both. Or, if you are having a nutritious wholefood cereal for breakfast, do not add bread to your morning carbohydrate intake as well.

Nutrigenomic research shows that humans thrive on a minimum of 650g of organically sourced vegetables each day. You cannot overeat or overdose on green leafy vegetables. We encourage you to include them at every meal.

GUIDELINE D

Eat slowly and not too much at each meal to support digestion.

Time-poor people rush their meals and eat too quickly. This means they often swallow lumps of food that are usually helped down by drinking water with food. The stomach is not designed to break down lumps of food; that is what our teeth are for.

Your stomach does not have teeth!

This means you need to chew each mouthful until the food is puree in your mouth before the next step of swallowing.

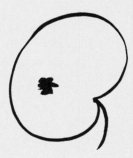

MINDFUL EATING

- Eat slowly and with care so you'll give your body the chance to digest and absorb the nutrients present in your meals.

- Think of your stomach as a baby: it can only cope with purees rather than a stir-fry.

- Meat requires more chewing than vegetables.

- Avoid water 20 minutes before, during and after eating to help improve digestion.

- Drink sufficient filtered water each day, just separate from meals.

- Drink 5ml of apple cider vinegar each morning – on an empty stomach – to help break down food (look for the 'mother' when purchasing).

- Apple cider vinegar may also help reduce heartburn or gastric reflux.

- Slowing down the rate you eat will also help reduce heartburn or gastric reflux.

- For good dental hygiene, rinse your mouth well with water after swallowing lemon juice or apple cider vinegar.

TOP TIP

Put your knife, fork or spoon down between each mouthful. Only pick up your cutlery once that mouthful has been chewed properly and swallowed.

GUIDELINE E

Follow the S.L.O.W food principle

The S.L.O.W food principle encourages us to eat whole, fresh food the way nature intended. S.L.O.W is an acronym for:

(S)EASONAL
(L)OCAL
(O)RGANIC
(W)HOLE

HOW TO GO SLOW

- Learn how to best stock your refrigerator and pantry. Pantry items should include spices, seasonings, whole grains, legumes, organic oils, vinegars and bottles of tomato puree. Limit food in cans. If you buy food in cans, ensure the tin lining is BPA-free (BPA is an endocrine-disrupting chemical). The lining is used as the internal seal to protect the can from the acidity of the food. Look inside any can and you will see there is a protective barrier between the can and the food.

- Wherever possible, buy at farmers' markets. You will be able to purchase what is in season, grown locally and it will generally have been picked in the last seven days.

- Develop a relationship with your local greengrocer and let it be known that pesticide-free, organic and fresh foods are important to you.

- Find a reliable supply of fresh, locally caught fish, if you live in coastal areas.

- If you eat meat, a good butcher is a godsend. Look for one who has an interest in grass-fed and organic meat and poultry.

- Grow your own veggies and herbs if you can. This 'living food' will lift your nutritional intake significantly. If you live in an apartment, use pots on your balcony or windowsill, or install a green wall. If you have a garden, convert one or two of your flower beds to grow food suitable for your climate and soil.

- Look into community gardens in your area – they're a great way to meet people and grow your own food.

ORGANIC FOOD: IS IT WORTH THE COST?

Our bodies are not designed to ingest residues of pesticides and herbicides. Chemicals such as these interfere with our microbiome, creating imbalances in our gut flora that affect our digestion (see You and Your Gut, page 123). Organic food can cost more, but food quality should be a priority as it is essential to good health and wellbeing.

Can't afford organic? Make a minimal investment in broccoli or leafy green items. Or grow your own.

Even a little bit of poison makes a big difference to your ability to reach a thriving state. Food advisory boards in Australia, New Zealand and the USA have not yet digested the emerging data coming from the research in the field of nutrigenomics. We cover this important concept in Chapter 12.

FOOD FACT

Over 80 per cent of the chemicals found in a human body come from conventionally farmed food sources.

Some of the chemicals found in conventionally farmed food sources are a contributor to the development of chronic disease such as diabetes, cardiovascular disease and cancer. Research has shown that pesticides sabotage the normal biochemical pathways in our body, which in turn interferes with many aspects of our health. Residual pesticides and herbicides are just another avoidable toxic burden on our body that can affect our ability to maintain a thriving state. Pesticides, herbicides and other chemicals such as chlorine and fluoride in our water supply can also impact the balance of our gut microbiome, our essential helper in all aspects of our optimal health.

HEALTH TIP

Drink only well-filtered water. Otherwise your body becomes the filter!

So how do you ensure you're eating as many fresh fruit and vegetables as possible, while avoiding these toxins? If buying organic produce is not an option for you, try farmers' markets and choose pesticide-free fruit and vegetables. Fruits, especially berries and leafy vegetables, are most vulnerable to pests and will be the most sprayed (resulting in higher levels of pesticide residue) so buying organic versions should be a priority.

KEEP IT CLEAN.

When buying non-organic produce, rinse well in vinegar and water before consuming. Use a mixture of around 1/2 cup (125ml) of vinegar to a litre of water.

WHICH FISH IS BEST?

Wherever possible, source your fish and seafood from clean waters from your own country or close by. In Australia, look for smaller fish that has been line-caught in Australian waters.

Try to avoid farmed fish. The concept is ideal for sustainability, but the reality is not yet perfect. In many fish farms, the stock is overfed food they are not designed to eat, over-medicated with antibiotics to prevent disease, and often overcrowded in their tanks and cages. It is good to see a movement in some fish farms to purge their fish of all antibiotics prior to releasing for sale; this is a good step in the right direction to produce a 'cleaner' product. Do your research, connect with your fish supplier (even if it is your supermarket). Hold them accountable to your questions and require your supplier to find out which fish farms are committed to doing a purge before sale.

If you shop well, you will eat well.

WHAT ARE WHOLE FOODS?

Whole foods are foods that have had little to no human intervention, such as meat, chicken, fish, fruit, vegetables and eggs. Supermarkets usually place whole foods in the outside aisles, kept refrigerated or cool. If a food item is packaged, this often indicates human interference. Buy the whole, real food item rather than the packaged version, and use food preparation techniques that can help retain its full nutritional value, such as steaming, baking and occasionally shallow-frying. Avoid overheating all oils and cooking fats and never allow any oils to smoke during cooking.

OILS TO USE FOR HEALTHIER COOKING:

- Olive oil if the heat is low (extra virgin is more heat stable).

- Walnut, macadamia oil and ghee are good for medium heat.

- Coconut oil and duck fat are very stable when high heat is required, but should only be used in small amounts or for celebratory occasions.

TO OIL OR NOT TO OIL?

Olive oil is a must in your diet. It's loaded with anti-inflammatory benefits for the arteries, brain and heart health. There is an abundance of evidence that this oil directly impacts gene function in a very positive way, explaining why some Mediterranean communities boast the longest-living residents on earth.

GUIDELINE F

You can still enjoy food freedom.

Have you heard of the 80:20 rule? It's a great way to balance out your healthy eating habits. By eating well (which means clean, healthful food) for 80 per cent of the time, you are following the 'Eat for Life' principles outlined here. For the remaining 20 per cent, you can live a little (but don't blow it completely!) For example, your 20 per cent can include a few slices of pizza, garlic bread and a glass of red wine.

One study found that you can lose weight by following the 80:20 rule, or, at the very least, you'd be healthier overall, and 'have a lower risk for conditions such as heart disease, high blood pressure and cancer'.

If you need to reduce body fat, your diet should be more restrictive (90:10 or even 100 per cent healthy) for a while. When you reach your goal weight, or are closer to it, you can return to the 80:20 rule.

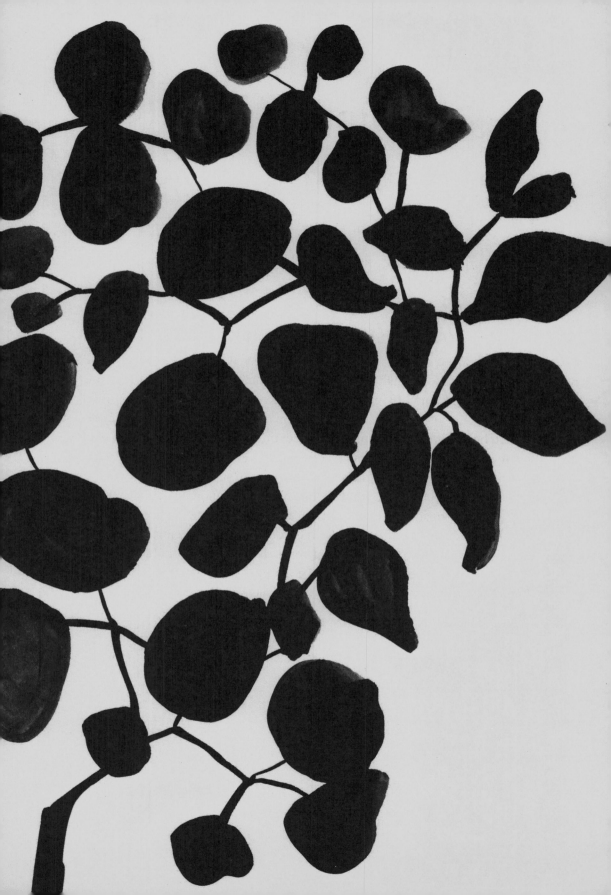

4.
YOU AND YOUR GUT

We are not
what we eat.
We are the
potential of
what we absorb.

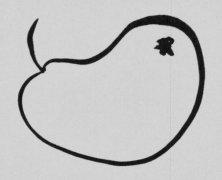

We believe that digestion and gut health is one of the most important aspects of our health and yet it tends to fly under the radar. Digestion refers to our body's ability to absorb nutrients and eliminate waste. It also influences if our body is burning or storing fat, building or losing muscle, creating or depleting energy and speeding or slowing the ageing process. Yet strangely enough, while everyone seems to have an opinion on what to eat (and what not to eat), few pay attention to the way their body processes the things they consume. You may be eating perfectly balanced, organic food and taking expensive supplements, but your body may only be absorbing a fraction of the available nutrients due to poor digestion.

WHAT'S YOUR GUT FEELING?

A major part of digestion is our gut integrity and gut bacteria. Our microbiome are the microscopic organisms that live in and on our body that help us to maintain health. We have approximately two kilograms of bacteria in our body. At the time of publishing this book, it is estimated that more than 5000 different species of friendly flora and over 100 trillion micro-organisms help us digest foods daily. It's pretty busy down there! The balance of 'good' and 'bad' gut bacteria is essential for many health outcomes in our life. A healthy gut produces vitamins B and K, enhances immunity and maintains pH balance. It also helps us metabolise pharmaceutical drugs, hormones and carcinogens, and ensures we have an abundance of energy.

Communication between the gut and our brain has more recently uncovered new research ground for neurologists to explore the significant relationship between Parkinson's disease, dementia and gut health.

Have you considered how any of these factors may affect your gut health?

COMPLETE THE AUDIT

HOW OFTEN DO YOU EXPERIENCE OR INGEST THE FOLLOWING?	NEVER	SOMETIMES	ALWAYS
Stress			
Processed food			
Fast food			
Sugar (which feeds the bad gut bacteria)			
Excessive table salt (more than one teaspoon of table salt)			
Antacids			
Herbicides and pesticides from non-organic foods			
Disrupted or insufficient sleep			
Ingested and transdermal chemicals (from non-organic skin care/household cleaning agents)			
Food intolerances			
Drugs			
Infection (for example, acute gastroenteritis, food poisoning or parasitic infections)			
Antibiotics			
Insufficient chewing			
Imbalanced diet (eating the same food every day or poor quality, low nutrient food)			
International travel			
Alcohol			
Excessive exercise			

If you tick three or more in the 'Always' column on this table, aim for improvement as you work your way through the chapters in this book.

LEAKY GUT

One of the common conditions affecting gut health and compromising digestion is leaky gut syndrome, also known as **compromised tight cell-wall junctions.**

The naturopathic community has been aware of the importance of gut wall integrity for decades and termed the condition 'leaky gut'. The use of this label was held in disdain by the medical fraternity. In 2009 the medical world 'discovered' an interesting observation on electron microscopy that they coined 'compromised tight cell-wall junctions'. And the existence of leaky gut was confirmed as a true medical condition.

Everything that enters the gut comes from the outside world. In a healthy gut, all macro and micronutrients from food are actively transported through the actual gut cells. These cells act as important gatekeepers and as a sponge exclusively for nutrients, keeping us safe from any harmful elements from the outside world. If these sponge-like cells become inflamed or damaged, spaces are created between these normally tightly bound cells.

This damage allows undigested food particles, microbes, toxins and wastes to slip through the intestinal wall and into the bloodstream, triggering a response from the white cell immune surveillance army. This excessive immune response may continue to feed inflammation in the gut wall over a period of days, months or even years. Naturopaths and Functional Nutritionists are in an ideal position to provide advice on how to manage and heal a leaky gut.

THE IMPORTANCE OF GUT HEALTH

Irritable Bowel Syndrome (IBS) and inflammatory bowel diseases like Ulcerative Colitis and Crohn's Disease are associated with an increased risk of dementia, highlighting the integral relationship between our gut and brain health as we age. This is why it is important to nurture the health of our gut and its microbiome.

Symptoms of leaky gut or impaired digestion include:

- reflux, heartburn, indigestion
- constipation, bloating, diarrhoea
- flatulence
- bad breath
- irritable bowel syndrome (IBS)
- dark circles under the eyes
- fatigue
- poor-quality hair, skin and nails
- puffiness
- fluid retention
- swollen glands
- joint pain
- increase in autoimmune disease
- anaemia
- unexplained weight gain/loss
- mood swings
- hormonal imbalances
- allergies such as sinus and hay fever
- skin conditions such as psoriasis and eczema

Needless to say, the effects of poor digestion can place great strain upon everyday life. Seek professional advice to determine the cause of any of the signs or symptoms listed here to eliminate significant medical disease as the cause.

HOW TO TREAT LEAKY GUT SYNDROME

Carolina Rossi, Registered Dietitian and Functional Nutritionist, says: 'If you have leaky gut syndrome, it's essential to heal it. Left unchecked, you will be missing out on essential nutrients and could also be exposing yourself to future complications that may become a serious health issue.'

Her recommendations are to remove the following from your diet for 30 days.

- Alcohol
- Sugar
- Processed food
- Gluten
- Dairy
- Soy
- Corn
- Eggs
- Fructose (including fruit juice) from your diet until your gut has healed

'After 30 days slowly introduce these foods into your diet, one-by-one. This will give your gut time to re-adjust to these foods, and you will also be able to take note to see if your gut reacts in some way to a specific food or food group,' says Rossi.

HEALING YOUR GUT WITH HERBS AND SUPPLEMENTS

Herbs and supplements can go a long way towards supporting your gut repair and digestive enzymes. Some to try include:

- aloe vera
- slippery elm
- glutamine
- probiotics
- selenium

- zinc
- copper
- manganese
- coenzyme Q10
- a good antioxidant complex

Some people respond well to aloe vera, for example, but for others it inflames the system. In cases of leaky gut, it would be wise to work with a naturopath to get you back in balance.

Naturopath Shannon McNeil shared with us her golden rules when it comes to eating to heal leaky gut syndrome. 'Herbs such as berberine and golden seal will also assist in healing the gut, along with the nutrients that Carolina suggests. It also helps to include healing foods such as ginger, garlic, turmeric, coconut milk, flaxseed, sauerkraut, kimchi, sprouted foods and warm broths in your daily diet. Boost your fibre intake by eating leafy greens, sweet potato, chia seeds and avocado to ensure you eliminate daily. Drink lots of filtered still water.'

FOOD INTOLERANCES AND ALLERGIES

The integrity of our gut can be challenged by food intolerances (the inability to digest a food) and allergies (a reaction by the immune system). However, at the same time, the health of our gut also protects us from developing food intolerances that may become a problem as we age or following an acute or chronic health condition or emotional overload. Allergies are generally caused by genetics or environmental factors.

Food intolerances vary according to the individual, but three of the most common are:

- gluten (found in many grains) and called non-coeliac gluten sensitivity by gastroenterologists

- casein (one of the proteins found in dairy)

- eggs (due to large proteins that are hard for the body to process)

If you suspect one of these food groups is the culprit, try avoiding all these foods for a month and then re-introduce them into your diet one at a time. It can be helpful to keep a record of what you eat and drink, and make note of any reactions, such as changes to your skin, bowel movements or energy levels, as well as how you feel after eating. Keep observing any signs or messages your body communicates to you for 48 hours after eating each reintroduced food.

In most instances, food intolerances can be improved with gut repair strategies and food avoidance under the guidance of a holistic or complementary practitioner, such as an integrated doctor, naturopath, holistic dietitian or nutritionist.

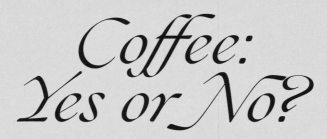

Coffee: Yes or No?

Could coffee be behind your stomach problems
(and the reason you have less than ideal sleep)?

How does your daily intake stack up?
Keep your caffeine intake to less than 100mg per day.

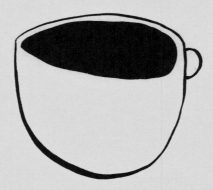

1 cup of brewed coffee = 95mg caffeine
1 espresso single shot = 65mg caffeine
100mg cocoa = 230mg caffeine

This could be the sole reason why you are not sleeping!

A SIX-WEEK LIVER CLEANSE FOR LIVER SUPPORT

The gut-liver connection is one of the most important partnerships in your body. Both need to be performing optimally to achieve a thriving state of being. The following strategies are designed to reduce liver loaders from the body for six weeks.

1.

Avoid any known food intolerances, like dairy or gluten.

2.

Choose organic where possible – this gives the liver a break from pesticide residues found in conventionally farmed food.

3.

In order for the liver detox to have the space and support it needs during this time, it's imperative that you cut out the following for six weeks:

No alcohol
No refined sugars
No caffeine

4.

Use the following supplements for a six-week liver cleanse:

- The herb St Mary's thistle containing 140mg of the active ingredient silymarin – take twice daily
- N-acetyl cysteine supplement 2g twice daily for six weeks only. This has been medically proven to be a powerful liver support nutrient. Avoid this if you have a history of kidney stones.
- Vitamin C 1000mg daily
- Slippery Elm Powder 7g daily

- Elemental magnesium 300mg daily

5.

Herbal teas can be added to the routine for a combination of hydration and liver support – dandelion tea is a good alternative to coffee while on the cleanse.

ONGOING LIVER SUPPORT STRATEGIES

After the six weeks, try to continue to minimise alcohol and caffeine. Check in with your body after re-introducing each product and be honest about the effect it has on your system.

HOW ANTACIDS CAN DO MORE HARM THAN GOOD

One little-known side effect of the antacid medication family – known as Proton Pump Inhibitors (like Nexium and Somac) – is the ability of these drugs to create havoc in the gut up to three weeks after you stop taking them.

While taking an antacid drug, stomach acid levels are pushed to much lower-than-natural acid concentrations. This can allow an appropriate time for an issue to heal, such as a gastric or duodenal ulcer. Once the healing process has resolved and the drug is stopped, a rebound hyperacidity can occur. This is where the level of acid temporarily jumps to high concentrations, mimicking symptoms identical to the original ulcer or reflux disease. The temptation is to hop straight back onto these meds in the mistaken belief that the underlying medical problem is still there.

Recent research on the dangers of long-term use of Proton Pump Inhibitors (PPIs) found a worrying link between an increased risk of 'all-cause mortality' (in other words, the risk of dying of all known medical diseases). This is likely due to the disruption of normal digestion caused by the long-term reduction of stomach acid and micronutrient nutritional deficiencies.

Discuss the solution to this dilemma with your health care professional.

RESTORING GUT MICROBIOME AFTER MEDICATION

If you require antibiotics (which can kill off good colonies from the gut), we suggest you introduce small amounts of fermented foods whilst you are taking your medication and continue to include these foods in your usual diet. This option is preferred to taking a course of practitioner-range probiotics. Recent research has shown that when compared with high-dose probiotics, good food choices can create a faster rebound of beneficial probiotics (while high-dose probiotics can delay re-colonisation for up to five months).

Ensure you support the newly introduced bacteria by reducing the number of gut disrupters you imbibe. These include alcohol, deep-fried foods and processed foods. Instead, eat foods that feed your gut. This includes fibre, beans and legumes as well as green leafy vegetables and fermented foods.

HEALTH NOTE

If you have had a course of chemotherapy, visit a complementary health practitioner (nutritional expert, naturopath or integrated doctor) who specialises in working alongside oncologists to re-establish gut integrity and the right bacterial culture in your gut.

PROBIOTIC TIPS

When sourcing a probiotic, look for one containing the family Saccharomyces Boulardii. This is a 'first coloniser' that will aid the establishment of other probiotic populations like lactobacillus and acidophilus. They provide the glue that makes other colonies stick to the gut wall.

A WORD ON ZINC

This essential mineral is a catalyst for over 84 different metabolic functions in your body, one of which is to assist in the production of hydrochloric acid in the stomach. Interestingly, if the hydrochloric acid in your stomach is low, your ability to absorb zinc from food is compromised, creating a cycle of chronic zinc deficiency.

To check your zinc levels, visit a naturopath or a health food store that offers naturopathic advice for a simple zinc tally test, or ask your doctor to do a blood test. It is essential that your body has an adequate supply of zinc to perform its many metabolic functions, such as building the immune system and supporting adrenal gland functions. Research on Covid-19 and similar viruses shows an increased risk of severe symptoms in those with low zinc levels. If your zinc levels are low, consider a practitioner-strength zinc supplement, rather than an over-the-counter sub-standard compound. These are best prescribed by your complementary health care professional.

THERE'S NO SUCH THING AS 'NORMAL'

The reference ranges for zinc levels vary from state to state and lab to lab. Strangely this is because the reference range in each state is calculated on population averages and can vary depending on your location. When we review the impact of zinc on health, we suggest the ideal reference range for serum zinc (regardless of where you live) should be between 14 and 28 micromol per litre.

YOUR 'NORMAL' ZINC RANGE MAY DIFFER TO WHAT YOUR PRACTITIONER TELLS YOU.

Ask for the number of your serum zinc when you get your results. If you are not within the 14–28 micromol per litre range, consider supplementation with the support of a good naturopath or integrative medical practitioner.

LOW ZINC? YOU MAY HAVE TOO MUCH COPPER

Good zinc levels are essential for optimal wellbeing. One of the saboteurs of good zinc levels in the body is copper.

Copper is also an essential mineral for good health, but too much of a good thing can cause a domino effect, resulting in the blockage of zinc absorption. If you struggle to increase and maintain good zinc levels despite supplementation, consider the possibility of copper overload.

There is one issue: zinc deficiency due to excess copper is usually resistant to standard zinc supplementation.

Copper overload is the most commonly encountered imbalance found on hair mineral testing. In essence, copper blocks zinc and other essential minerals from functioning in their normal biochemical pathways of wellness. This can create a cascade of poor health that can start at birth. Copper can pass over the placenta to create a zinc deficiency state from birth in some babies whose mothers are both copper overloaded and zinc deficient. This may also result in common conditions like gastric reflux and colic in the newborn.

SIGNS OF COPPER OVERLOAD

FATIGUE

MENSTRUAL DISORDERS

HEAVY PERIODS

PMS

INFERTILITY

DEPRESSION

ANXIETY

MIGRAINES

ALLERGIES

CHILDHOOD LEARNING DISORDERS

CAUSE OF COPPER OVERLOAD

The use of copper cookware, copper plumbing, herbicide sprays of copper sulphate on vegetables and in the water supply all contribute to an excess availability of copper. The oral contraceptive pill can also contribute to copper overload.

HOW TO DO A COPPER 'DUMP'

Certain foods have been used traditionally as copper chelators (binding agents). Increase parsley, garlic and coriander in your diet as these foods can bind with excess copper and help you eliminate it efficiently. The trace mineral molybdenum helps the liver remove copper and is abundant in foods that grow above the ground, like beans, peas, broccoli and cabbage. Selenium-rich foods like brazil nuts can also help to regulate copper levels.

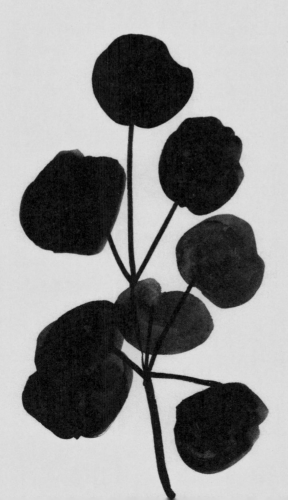

ELIMINATION

The last step in the digestion process is elimination. With bowel cancer on the rise and other digestive issues such as colitis, haemorrhoids, constipation and appendicitis affecting a large portion of the population, it is worth reviewing your toilet habits (no need to be prim!).

Bowel cancer is the third most common type of newly diagnosed cancer in Australia.

Our colon is six feet long and stores all our waste. As the waste moves towards the rectum, the puborectalis muscle chokes the rectum to maintain continence.

In a sitting position, the puborectalis muscle is only partially relaxed. However in a deep squat position this muscle is fully relaxed and allows waste to be completely eliminated. The modern toilet is an invention borne of convenience and luxury, rather than science. The truth is, squatting is the way humans are anatomically designed to remove their waste.

SOLUTIONS TO IMPROVE YOUR ELIMINATION

- Consider buying a device like the 'Squatty Potty' (a footstool that nestles in front of your toilet) so you can raise your feet into the ideal position to release the puborectalis muscle. This is a simple and easy way to improve your elimination daily.

- Epsom salts is a safe and natural support for constipation. The suitable dose varies from person to person. Try a level teaspoon dissolved in black tea at bedtime and increase by ½ teaspoon daily until you achieve the desired effect. This product is pure magnesium sulphate and has other health benefits on top of its ability to improve transit time in the large intestine. These include muscle relaxation, improved sleep quality and subtle mood benefits.

- Aloe vera juice can work wonders for some people but take care as it can be an irritant for a minority.

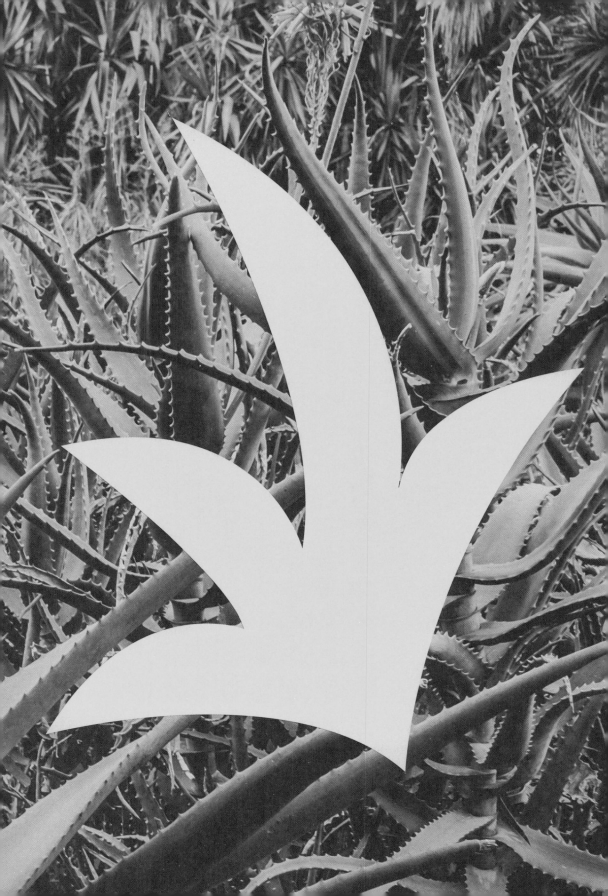

ALOE VERA JUICE RECIPE

This is a favourite recipe from Gwinganna Lifestyle Retreat's organic gardener Shelley Pryor. Make sure you use the large-leaf aloe barbadensis plant, which has more potent medicinal qualities.

1   Use a leaf approximately 20cm long and 6cm wide – the size of a small fish.

2   Fillet the leaf, removing all of the green outer rind on both sides. You will be left with a clear gel inner fillet.

3   Cut this fillet into pieces around 6–8cm wide (3–4 inches).

4   Wash these in clean water for a few seconds to remove some of the outer slime.

5   Fill a 2L container with clean filtered water.

6   Add the rinsed fillets to the container and refrigerate for 8 hours before first use.

7   Recommended dose is ½ cup (125ml) of aloe juice infusion twice daily.

8   After removing each ½ cup of aloe for use, add ½ cup of water back into the container so that it always holds 2L. This remains potent in the fridge for around seven days.

9   Discard after seven days and restart the process.

HOW TRAVEL CAN AFFECT YOUR GUT HEALTH

If travelling overseas, the change in time zones will interfere with your circadian rhythm, which may disrupt the balance of bacteria in your gut. Take a four-week course of probiotics before you leave and, for best results, another course during your trip then repeat for four weeks after you return home. Try and rotate through different brands of probiotics as they will deliver different families of good bacteria.

International travel could mean you may be exposed to parasites that can go undetected for years and are often not diagnosed until serious symptoms show up. They can play havoc with our gut and digestion. Most naturopaths are very adept at eliminating parasites with an elimination diet and herbal remedies. If you feel unwell on return from overseas, you should seek advice from your health professional. If travelling to countries where you will be exposed to unsafe water and lower food hygiene standards, take probiotics with you and drink fresh turmeric and ginger teas whenever possible. These potent roots have anti-inflammatory properties and can act as a deterrent to any parasite infection. Grate or finely chop them and infuse in boiling water, then drink hot or cold throughout the day. Hotel staff can tell you where to find these ingredients or may even get them for you.

GUT HEALTH SOLUTIONS

General strategies for maintaining a healthy gut

- Sip an infusion of hot lemon, fresh turmeric and ginger tea upon rising each morning to help alkalise your body. It can be cooled to room temperature if you prefer.

- Ten minutes before breakfast (and other meals if digestion is poor), take one teaspoon of raw apple cider vinegar neat, or in a little water to help your stomach acid effectively digest food. (The apple cider vinegar must contain the 'mother').

- Eat organic food (remember pesticide and herbicide residue interfere with gut bacteria and can create and exacerbate a leaky gut).

- Gradually include a small amount of fermented foods in your diet as tolerated, such as miso, sauerkraut, kimchi and tamari. Remember that more is not necessarily better!

- Eat plentiful pesticide-free vegetables and green leafy foods.

- Chew food until it has the consistency of puree before swallowing, and pause after each mouthful to allow the food to reach your stomach before you put another forkful into your mouth.

- Avoid over-eating. Two fistful-sized amounts of food – one of protein and one of carbohydrates, plus green leafy vegetables – should be the maximum you eat per meal. Around 25 to 30 per cent of your meal should come from whole fats.

- Drink 2–3 litres of filtered still water each day.

- Keep your caffeine intake to less than 100mg per day. Be aware of hidden caffeine in foods like cacao used in chocolate.

- Avoid alcohol, or at least have three to four alcohol-free days each week. Stay within the recommended daily intake of one to two standard drinks when you do drink. See opposite page for standard drink measurements.

- Avoid drinking while eating and for 20 minutes before and after a meal. One glass of (ideally) red wine during a meal can aid digestion in people with a healthy gut, but check with your nutritional expert first.

- Make sure you get seven to eight hours of quality sleep each night.

- If you live with a lot of pressure (even if you manage it well), consider taking a practitioner-range probiotic every night. It's recommended that you rotate brands to ensure you replenish different probiotic families. Take a probiotic break for a month every six weeks to give your gut a chance to recalibrate.

- Check your zinc levels (health food shops and some pharmacies often offer their customers naturopathic testing for zinc status) and take a supplement if low.

- Avoid antacids – they reduce stomach acid, which reduces the body's ability to break down food particles. This affects our ability to digest food. The eventual side effect of antacids may be reduced nutrient absorption, leading to more gut health issues (more info on page 134).

WHAT IS A STANDARD DRINK?

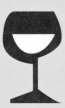

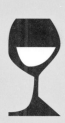

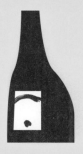

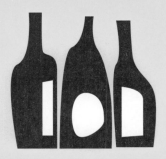

White Wine
Half a glass
1.4 standard drinks
11.5% alcohol
150 ml average serving

Red Wine
Half a glass
1.5 standard drinks
13% alcohol
150 ml average serving

Wine
750 ml bottle
6-8 standard drinks
11-13% alcohol

Wine
2 litre cask of wine
18-21 standard drinks
11-13% alcohol

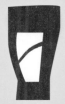

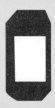

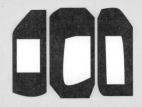

Beer (Full strength)
285 ml glass (middy)
1.1 standard drinks
4.8% alcohol

Beer (Full strength)
425 ml glass (schooner)
1.6 standard drinks
4.8% alcohol

Beer (Full strength)
375 ml can
1.4 standard drinks
4.8% alcohol

Beer (Full strength)
24 × 375 ml cans
34 standard drinks
4.8% alcohol

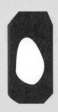

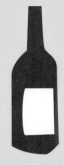

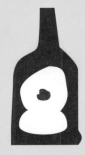

Spirits (High strength)
30 ml nip (shot glass)
1 standard drink
40% alcohol

Spirits (Ready to drink)
375 ml (premix can)
1.5 standard drinks
5% alcohol

Spirits (Ready to drink)
660 ml (large premix bottle)
3.6 standard drinks
7% alcohol

Spirits (High strength)
700 ml spirit bottle
22 standard drinks
40% alcohol

Gut solutions

Depending on your current State of Being, here are further tips to improve your gut health.

DEPLETED STATE OF BEING

If you are currently in a Depleted State of Being, it is highly likely that your digestion and gut integrity has been compromised. Without effective digestion it will be challenging for your body to heal itself. Like all living organisms, humans need nutrients and without these building blocks our body can simply not repair itself.

Eat cooked, rather than raw food for a while. This is a traditionally gut-supporting way of eating. Think about the difference between home-made chicken soup as opposed to a leaf of lettuce and an organic carrot. Both are healthy options, but warm food is much easier to process when your State of Being is depleted. If you have been under pressure due to emotional upheaval, strong pharmaceutical regimes and/or chronic illness, it is highly likely your digestive tract and gut microbiome will need restoration. Your body needs lots of nourishment during this time, and ensuring it can absorb good food is an essential step in your recovery. Gut recovery is best achieved when working in partnership with a qualified nutrition expert.

Seek a diagnosis from a naturopath, nutritional expert or integrative doctor as soon as possible.

SURVIVING STATE OF BEING

If you believe you are in a Surviving State of Being, your digestion is under threat. Follow the advice in this chapter to improve your digestion and seek professional advice if you have any concerns. Cut out alcohol and caffeine for a while until you are restored to thriving. Take time out for yourself; see healthy boundaries on page 218 for some strategies.

Many people in this state believe they know a lot about food and feel they are eating a balanced diet. Most are overlooking some essential pieces to the puzzle. Always include some fermented foods in your diet. Nutrition is an important step towards thriving, so pay close attention to how your meals stack up. Survivors are often prone to eating on the run, skipping meals or cutting out food groups to keep weight under control, and/or adopting fad diets. Sometimes they have beliefs about food that literally put their bodies into a stress response state. People in this group often experience some food allergies or intolerances that are usually the result of a compromised gut and digestive system. Review the way you eat every day and if anything feels unbalanced, make your nutritional needs a major priority in your life. A qualified nutritional expert can help you improve your body's ability to absorb nutrients.

THRIVING STATE OF BEING

If you know you feel great all the time and you believe you have the food formula right, this chapter is simply reinforcement of your way of living. However, we encourage you to read it carefully as you may still be able to improve your food choices and gut health to ensure you continue to thrive. Be aware of times of high stress that can hijack the digestive processes.

If you are currently in a Thriving State of Being, a major part of you staying in this state is taking care of your digestion. Pay close attention to your bowel movements and take action if you notice any gut symptoms or change in digestion and bowel habits.

Take a breath.

As we embark
on Pillar Two...

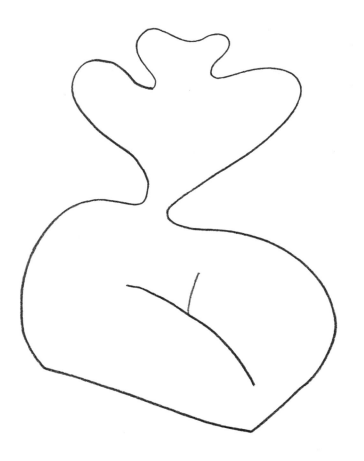

5.
FUNCTIONAL MOVEMENT AND EXERCISE

The less you move
on the ground, the
more the world
moves around.

ANA CLAUDIA ANTUNES
THE TAO OF PHYSICAL AND SPIRITUAL

SHARON
Oh what a feeling!
How our approach to fitness
has changed since the '80s.

'In the year 1980, my fitness career was born. For the next decade
and a half my life was a kaleidoscope of headbands, leg warmers and
fluorescent lycra. Exercising to music in classes (known as aerobics) was
almost *de rigueur*, promoted and popularised by celebrities such as Jane
Fonda and Olivia Newton-John. Lycra became acceptable streetwear for
me and many others of my generation. Considering it was on-trend to wear
a G-string leotard *over* tights, I think all that bouncing about must have
loosened a few screws!'

DR KAREN
The rise of the 'Superwoman'.

'The 1980s was a decade of inappropriate work/life balance for me.
I graduated from university in 1982 and started a torturous internship at
Royal Canberra Hospital. Newly married, I juggled competition squash,
scuba diving and cross-country skiing with an 80-hour working week.
In retrospect, some yoga or Pilates would have been a better choice; but
it was the '80s where women were told they could "have it all". We didn't
dwell on the consequences of hard physical activity until it was time to
have babies. I think my generation was the first to suffer the effects of
adrenal exhaustion and stress. This is what today in this book, we call
a Depleted State of Being.'

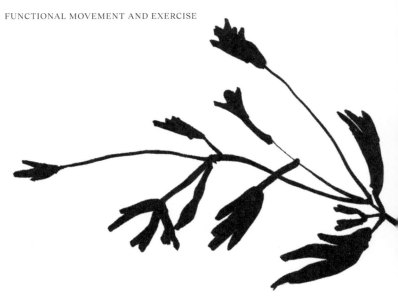

Before the craze for all things aerobic – which began in the '70s – it was rare for anyone other than athletes to perform endurance (aerobic) exercise, let alone the types of actions and movements required in an aerobics class. But aerobic exercise was taken up with gusto, along with lifting weights, jogging and yoga. Fitness was becoming a multi-billion-dollar industry that would give rise to enormous amounts of guilt in millions of people. However, the merits of too much of this type of exercise are now very much in question.

Today, we are beginning to understand the truth about our body's physical needs. While stimulating the cardiovascular system is important, we are learning that excessive sustained, intense aerobic exercise can be detrimental to our heart, blood vessels, skeleton, joints, muscles and immune system.

We asked Jason Kaplan, physician and preventive cardiologist, about his thoughts on excessive, intense exercise in relation to our heart, brain and arterial health. How much is excessive and what are the concerns?

DR JASON KAPLAN, MD,
SPECIALIST CARDIOLOGIST AND PHYSICIAN

Are you over-exercising?

Hippocrates said that 'Everything in excess is opposed to nature'. I believe 'exercise is medicine' and is in fact one of the most beneficial lifestyle interventions we can do. However, there may be issues relating to underdosing and overdosing. There is a U-shaped curve between running 'doses' and all-cause mortality: once participants get beyond three hours of vigorous running per week, there is little additive cardiovascular benefit, and if this is exceeded significantly, there may be harmful effects.

Our society (first-world countries) has, overall, a problem of lack of exercise, as opposed to an excess of movement. However, there is around two to five per cent of the population who may be overdoing exercise training and causing subtle cardiac damage. This cardiac damage may include fibrosis of the heart muscle, an excess of calcification in the arteries in some endurance athletes, and the development of certain heart arrhythmias. Despite this, cardiovascular aerobic fitness is one of the strongest predictors of longevity. Above-average activity for one's age should be a goal for people who would like to increase life expectancy.

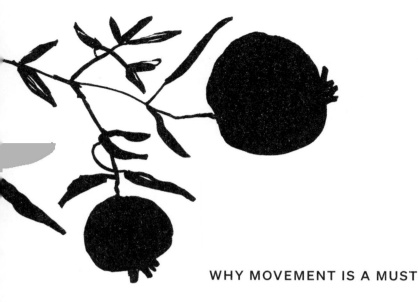

WHY MOVEMENT IS A MUST

There is a staggering amount of research that shows a sedentary lifestyle is detrimental to all of our body systems and leads to a decrease in human health. Our bodies are designed to be active and to move regularly, so we can stimulate muscle, bone density, nerve health and vascular dilation regularly. Whilst cardiovascular fitness is a major contributing factor to our health, what is essential, and if not more important, is our physical function. This means ensuring our muscles, bones and nervous system interact in a way that allows us to perform regular daily tasks, like getting in and out of a car, carrying children, or picking up something from the floor without injury. Having joints that work through a full range of movement without pain will make a difference to our mental and emotional state as well as our ability to stay active in life, within the bounds of individual physical limitations.

The word 'exercise' conjures up mental pictures of running, spinning or cycling. You're not alone if you think these forms of exercise are the Holy Grail. Younger people, and those who are biomechanically sound, can enjoy these activities in moderation. For many though, these activities can increase inflammation in the body, place excessive pressure on joints and increase the long-term stress hormone cortisol. These kinds of activities may be creating problems rather than assisting health. Just like a nutritional diet, the prescription for exercise should be based on an individual's genetic, physical and biochemical make up and the body's current State of Being.

WHY RUNNING MAY NOT BE THE HOLY GRAIL

You may have noticed that people who choose marathons and endurance sports as their chosen exercise routine can look older than their chronological age.

If you've always run or competed in marathons, we applaud you. However, as you get older you may find that you don't recover as quickly, or your body may be sending you messages to slow down in the form of joint pain, acute injuries or even a diagnosis of osteoarthritis. It may be that your body is suffering from an increase of inflammation driven by an excessive stress-hormone response.

When you run at high intensity for extended periods of time, your body's interpretation of this activity is that you are in danger. It then produces stress hormones to assist you to run or fight in order to save your life. Whilst you are not in danger when competing in a marathon or running, the ancient pathways will still become activated. And the increase in stress hormones, particularly cortisol, accelerates the ageing process.

Cortisol also inhibits your body's capacity to burn fat as an energy source. Interestingly, cortisol is a major culprit in fat/weight gain. If the primary goal is to reduce or maintain body fat levels, excessive running and cycling may not the best or only way to achieve this goal. It depends on the individual.

TO LIFT OR NOT TO LIFT?

Keeping muscle mass high will drive your metabolic rate up. This is how we burn most of our calories. The more muscle you have, the bigger your motor. Think of a four-cylinder car and how much fuel it takes. Now think of a V8 and how much more fuel it needs to drive the same distance. This is just the start of what our muscle mass – the unsung hero – can do for our health. We encourage you to shift your perspective. When you think of the word exercise, consider it a mechanism via which you can grow your muscle mass. This will ensure you maintain joint stability, bone density, nerve function and so much more. Since muscles need a lot of blood flow, when you do a really good muscle workout you also meet the needs of the cardiovascular system. Exercise activities like weight training, Pilates and yoga can get your heart rate up sufficiently when you perform certain movements. It's a win-win.

Movement and exercise effect two primary things in your body. Primal movement patterns keep your body fully functional, while fine motor skills stimulate your brain. Any movement or exercise that generates these two essential outcomes will guarantee you will develop strength, stability, flexibility, mobility and agility. Performed regularly, it will also ensure you retain these qualities as you age.

PRIMAL MOVEMENTS

Evolution has bestowed innate patterns of movement upon us. Californian Clinical exercise specialist Paul Chek identified seven key actions, calling them 'primal pattern' movements.

During your childhood, you probably performed them daily; yet for those of us in the Western world, doing these movements become more and more infrequent as you get older. It's important to reverse this trend, as these patterns of movement are key to ensure you age with fully functioning physicality, allowing you to dance, pick up your grandchildren, and maintain shape and function.

Any movement you perform is comprised of one or more of seven primal pattern movements. These are:

1   Squatting e.g. going to the toilet, sitting down
2   Lunging e.g. stepping onto the bus
3   Bending e.g. picking something up from the floor
4   Twisting e.g. looking behind you
5   Pushing e.g. closing the car boot
6   Pulling e.g. opening a door
7   The gait cycle e.g. any motion where you transfer weight from one foot to the next, such as walking, jogging and sprinting

Humans have been reliant on these actions for their very survival throughout history. As Palaeolithic hunter-gatherers, we performed these actions for hours and hours, every single day. In those times, if we were unable to perform these movements we simply couldn't survive. The homo-sapien design of our bodies hasn't changed, so these actions are equally important in today's world, regardless of how different our lives may be. Exercise such as yoga, Pilates and functional movement classes consist entirely of primal pattern movements and give exceptional benefits when practiced regularly and safely.

FINE MOTOR SKILLS AND OUR BRAIN

There is a growing body of evidence reinforcing the need to maintain and improve fine motor skills throughout our life, as they support – and may improve – mental function. The areas of your brain that are related to movement and co-ordination need stimulation in order to optimally perform mental challenges and problem-solving. Activities that involve balancing and coordination also reduce the potential for mental deterioration and neurological disorders as you mature. Try juggling or balancing on a wobble board or do some of your daily activities with your non-dominant hand (try using your computer mouse, brushing your teeth or hair, stirring pots, or writing with the hand you don't usually use) to challenge these capacities. The benefits are greater mental acuity, focus and powers of concentration, so don't give up too easily!

When you challenge yourself, either physically (by learning how to perform a new movement, for instance) or mentally (learning a new language or musical instrument), fresh neurons and synapses are created in your brain. These adaptations are made possible by the brain's plastic and mutable nature, often referred to as its neuroplasticity.

The fun we all had playing games in the schoolyard, playground, park, backyard and on the beach as children, before the age of technology, taught your body to catch, throw, react, reflex and balance. Games like hopscotch, sevens (throwing a ball against a wall in different ways), handball, elastics, Simon says, British bulldogs and French cricket all helped your development in various ways. Reproducing some of these games, particularly as you get older, stimulates the brain in a positive way. Next time you're out with your children or grandchildren, introduce them to these games if they don't know them. Don't just sit and watch them play – join in, and you will all benefit.

MOVING OUR BODIES

Many people under-exercise, many people over-exercise, but most people simply 'under-move'. There are few people who have hit that sweet spot and get the balance right.

ARE YOU AN 'UNDER-MOVER'?

The under-moving group includes a lot of over-exercisers. Yes, you heard right; those over-exercising addicts generally don't move enough. How could that be, you ask? Think about it. They go flat out when it's 'exercise time', but for the rest of the day they don't feel the need to move because they believe they've fulfilled their exercise quota. They may be virtually inert for the rest of the day. Research is emerging that shows regular movement all day is more beneficial than cramming a lot of movement into one little chunk.

Performing thousands of small movements throughout the day is what's most beneficial for our health.

The story of exercising and moving is therefore a two-part tale – that of moving and that of exercising. They sound one and the same, but they are really quite distinct.

This makes moving fundamental to our nature, and exercising circumstantial. Moving is what we must do regularly and abundantly, whilst exercising is what we should do regularly, but not to excess.

KARL OSTROWSKI,
HUMAN MOVEMENT SPECIALIST BHM (HONS) AND RESEARCHER

Constant Intermittent Movement [CIM]

CIM is the singular most important aspect of how we should move our bodies. It should occur throughout the day, until we switch off at night. However, many of us are simply not doing it. Historically, our ancestors performed CIM every day, from sunrise till sunset. CIM is crucial to avoid the body breaking down and degenerating as you mature. CIM is also vital to your continued ability to move with competence, efficiency, economy and grace. Furthermore, CIM plays a pivotal role in immune function and, consequently, the prevention of disease.

Without CIM, there is an acceleration in the degeneration of the various systems of your body as you get older. The obvious systems that CIM supports are those that contain nerves, muscles, bones and joints. But systems that involve lymph fluid, digestion, immunity, respiration, hormones and circulation are just as reliant on CIM to function smoothly. Consequently, performing CIM is absolutely vital for hormonal balance, disease prevention, effective digestion, regular breathing and adequate circulation.

The instrument most responsible for the dramatic decline in CIM over the past 200 years is the chair. An office worker typically spends six hours sitting in an eight-hour workday. The time spent sitting in transit and sitting at home adds additional hours. Some people spend as much as 12 hours a day sitting.

How detrimental is all this sitting to your health? A British study examining 4512 people over four years found that those who spent more than four hours per day sitting in front of a TV or computer screen were twice as likely to be hospitalised or suffer a major cardiac episode. This was compared to those who spent less than two hours before a screen.

And an American study showed that those in sitting occupations were 54 per cent more likely to suffer a heart event than those whose job had them on their feet. An Australian study observing 200,000 subjects over three years demonstrated that sitting for 11 hours or more per day resulted in a 40 per cent greater chance of dying, than those who spent less than four hours per day sitting. These results are shocking and reinforce the fact that we were born to be moving. In essence, we need to be performing CIM.

There are a host of physical consequences when sitting:

1   Lymphatic circulation ceases, as lymph fluid cannot flow through the lymphatic pathways without muscular contraction.

2   Without the lymphatic system operating, immune function and fat metabolism are compromised so the potential for plaque build-up and other heart disease factors is exacerbated.

3   Sitting causes an increase in blood glucose levels and a pronounced drop in calorie expenditure, leading to increased body fat.

4   Sitting causes blood pools in veins and this can result in circulatory issues such as varicose veins and DVT, as well as adding to the risk of heart disease risk factors, like atherosclerosis.

5   Sitting also affects the pelvic floor. When you stand or squat, the pelvic floor develops a resting tension or tone, but when you are seated it becomes disengaged. As bladder control is related to pelvic floor control, excessive sitting increases risk for incontinence. What's more, the immobility imposed by sitting contributes to lamination, or sticking together and stiffening, of the muscles and tendons throughout the back and hips. All that sitting increases the likelihood of back pain and discomfort - not to mention spinal deterioration.

Regular movement supports the efficiency of more than 4000 helpful genes in our body.

SIMPLE SOLUTIONS TO HELP YOU MOVE MORE

There are some readers who may be challenged by a medical condition that limits exercise. This could be heart, lung, injury or disability related. There is overwhelming research that shows performing physical activity will improve your quality of life, lift a low mood and help with pain management. It will also extend your life span.

For any woman who feels she falls into this challenged category we recommend sourcing an appropriate 'coach'. Physiotherapy, Pilates and the emerging field of Exercise Physiology are all a good starting point for anyone with chronic medical conditions. These professionals can be found through a referral from your local doctor and visits are often covered by private medical insurance.

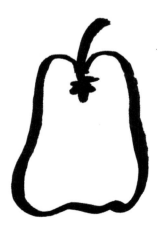

CASE STUDY | DR KAREN

Lynne

Persistence in the face of significant medical obstacles

My patient Lynne was a 64-year-old woman who had been fit and active, attending gym and walking regularly to keep fit. She had been diagnosed with Bradycardia (a slow heartbeat) due to an electrical problem with her heart, requiring a pacemaker. After her heart scare, she had upped the exercise in line with research that says exercise is great cardiovascular medicine.

She consulted me after she had seen her cardiologist for the annual check-up of her pacemaker, and we were both shocked to hear that her specialist had advised her to stop all physical activity! The story behind this unusual advice started with a review of her pacemaker leads from the pacing device to her heart muscle. The exercises she was doing had caused a premature shearing and wearing of the wires as they travelled across the left side of her upper chest.

Not satisfied with the situation, she sought my advice on how to maintain her fitness and keep her cardiologist happy. With the help of an exercise physiologist I was able to approve a good movement program that limited some minor movement of the left shoulder area and protected the pacemaker wires, but kept the rest of her body fit and strong. This solution was a win-win for her heart and health.

The same principles apply if you are injured or have limited mobility for medical reasons. Unless there are serious limitations to your physical body, there is nearly always a way to maintain your participation in the foundations of good movement.

HOW TO BUILD MORE MOVEMENT INTO YOUR DAILY ROUTINE

- Alternate standing and sitting at your desk – use the opportunity to physically move from one position to another. Remember, good posture is key in both sitting and standing.

- Use computer ergonomics software, such as 'WorkPace', which monitors and generates breaks in your work day and stimulates movement via regulated prompts. Or schedule your own breaks without the software by setting an alarm on your computer, watch or smartphone.

- Invest in a fitness tracker, such as Apple Watch or Fitbit, to record and report your incidental movement throughout the day. Aim for 8000-10,000 steps a day. Health benefits of regular movement kicks in when you're consistently charting a minimum of 7000 steps each day.

SIX SIMPLE WAYS TO INCREASE YOUR DAILY STEPS

1   Take the stairs as often as possible – see this as an opportunity and view escalators, lifts and conveyors as a last resort.

2   At the shopping centre, park your car as far away from the shops you need to visit as possible.

3   If you are physically sound and able-bodied with no back complaints, carry a basket when you shop and avoid using a trolley (within reason).

4   If you are physically sound and able-bodied, go for a walk at lunchtime, even if it's just a quick trip around the block.

5   Make movement a priority in your life; look for opportunities to move more.

6   Play with your children and pets in a physically active way.

Why over-exercising can be bad for you

If you are a regular exerciser and love to push your cardio, before you put this book down, pause and consider reading further to make sure you are hitting the sweet spot of ideal exercise.

Do the following audit to find out whether you are pushing your stress hormone pathways by over-exercising. If you regularly exercise, have you experienced:

COLDS AND FLUS
FOOD ALLERGIES
DIGESTIVE DISORDERS
MENSTRUAL IMBALANCES
ANXIETY
SLEEPLESS NIGHTS
INJURIES AND PERSISTENT PAIN

Too much exercise pushes muscles into the lactic acid zone in order to produce the energy required. This means that muscles produce more free radicals, which in turn increases inflammation in the body.

When you perform intense exercise too often and for too long, you put your system under strain. Pushing beyond your sweet spot into over-exercise suppresses your immune system. Digestion becomes compromised and the ability to absorb nutrients from food diminishes. The adrenal glands are overworked, undernourished and become stressed. This can manifest in chronic fatigue.

Good health for you may lie in more restorative 'Yin' movements such as Yoga, Qi Gong, Pilates, and walking. Most importantly it is the CIM (Continuous Intermittent Movement) that is the key factor in your health and wellbeing, particularly in your ability to manage your muscle, bone, fat, and fluid balance.

Do you need to do more 'Yin' (e.g. Yoga, moving meditation, Pilates, dance or gentle walking) or 'Yang' (e.g. spinning, boxing, interval training or weight training)? The answer depends on your current State of Being. The answer will also change as we move through our fertile years into our 40s, and through to the menopause and beyond.

FOCUS ON STRENGTH

Maintaining our strength is of primary importance, regardless of your **State of Being**. It becomes the first step in physical recovery from a depleted state.

The best activities are those that require your body to use the primal pattern movements mentioned earlier. Muscles are vital for maintaining a robust metabolism, controlling blood sugar levels and balancing hormones. They are responsible for at least 60 per cent of our resting metabolic rate, which is an enormous portion of the overall energy your body burns. If your body loses muscle, you require less energy to exist. This means that all the energy not used by muscles stores as fat.

Exercise that builds and maintains muscle is vital as you age. It is useful to do this sort of exercise even before the age of 30, because this is how we maintain bone density and increase our metabolism to manage our body composition (proportion of fat-to-muscle ratio). Using your body weight to push against gravity is the basis of challenging your muscles – your muscles adapt, and you get stronger. Yoga, Pilates, and lifting weights in a functional manner are the best exercises to improve your body as you age. If you have physical limitations, swimming, deep-water running and other water-based exercise options are your friend, as are Pilates sessions led by a physiotherapist. If you have arthritis, it is essential to move your joints and keep your muscles strong. Weak muscles put more strain on your damaged joints because they aren't supporting them sufficiently.

Before you book yourself into a course of something like CrossFit or any other intense group workout method, take stock of your adrenal system by noting your daily energy levels, and auditing your sleep patterns.

If energy levels are low and your sleep patterns are irregular, visit a naturopath for review of your adrenal system (see our Resources section for some suggestions). Exercise stimulates the adrenal glands, so if your system is already overstressed, it's best to opt for restorative Yin exercise until you're back on track.

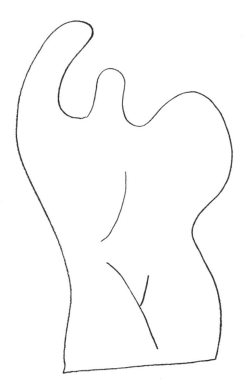

SOLUTIONS AND SUGGESTIONS

Which exercise is best for you at your present state?

DEPLETED STATE OF BEING

Your approach to exercise needs to support the adrenal system while it replenishes, so choose restorative styles of exercise to promote healing. Restorative yoga is amazing for adrenal support and also allows your body to rest in poses that assist your posture and decrease joint, neck and back pain. Find a teacher who has studied the correct approach to restorative yoga.

Strength and flexibility: aim for two to three Yin movement sessions a week and include some of the following options:

YIN OR RESTORATIVE YOGA **QI GONG/TAI CHI**
STRETCH CLASS **GENTLE PILATES**

Limit aerobic or cardiovascular training to just five minutes once or twice a week and slowly increase as your health improves. Consider the following options:

POWER WALKING **SWIMMING**
DEEP WATER RUNNING

SURVIVING STATE OF BEING

Being psychologically stressed and then overstressing the body with exercise is a recipe for disaster. A stressed body produces higher levels of cortisol, which can reduce the body's ability to burn fat and increase fat storage. If fat reduction is a goal, over-exercising is not the answer.

Many women are surprised to learn that during a busy day, the adrenals may be silently overworking. Over time these glands become stressed and depleted. Too much Yang exercise will exacerbate this problem. Once your body is thriving and the adrenal glands are fully functioning you can increase more Yang exercise. For now, ensure you have CIM in your life and approach your exercise component with an intention to support your body to be healthy.

Aim for three to four exercise sessions per week. Remember to balance your Yin and Yang activities.

YIN ACTIVITIES TO INCLUDE:

TAI CHI	YIN YOGA
QI GONG	PILATES AND STRETCHING

YANG ACTIVITIES TO INCLUDE:

IYENGAR OR ASHTANGA YOGA	WEIGHT TRAINING
INTERVAL TRAINING IN THE WATER	BOXING
OR ON LAND	SHORT DISTANCE AND INTERVAL
ROWING	RUNNING
CYCLING	

THRIVING STATE OF BEING

Listening to the messages your body is sending every day is an essential element to maintaining a Thriving State. When we are truly feeling fabulous on all levels, sleeping soundly and experiencing an abundance of energy, exercising intensely feels wonderful. However, remember more is not better. CIM should also be a foundation for all movement options. Follow the recommendations below and you will stay on track.

A word of caution: there will be times when life is throwing curve balls. At these times you may need to back off and reduce the intensity of your workouts. Knowing your body and understanding its needs is paramount and no amount of drive should influence your intuition about your body's State of Being.

Aim for three to five exercise sessions per week and remember to balance your Yin and Yang activities.

YIN ACTIVITIES TO INCLUDE:

TAI CHI

QI GONG

YIN YOGA

PILATES AND STRETCHING

YANG ACTIVITIES TO INCLUDE:

IYENGAR OR ASHTANGA YOGA

INTERVAL TRAINING IN THE WATER

OR ON LAND

ROWING

CYCLING

WEIGHT TRAINING

SPINNING

BOXING

RUNNING

THE HEALTH BENEFITS OF SPORTS AND HOBBIES

Getting involved in additional activities that allow you to be with like-minded people who you share a passion with is a healthy addition to your exercise regime. Gardening, bushwalking, horse-riding, playing tennis, sailing and rowing are all good examples. Remember to keep the balance and still focus on CIM.

If you participate in sports that require frequent use of one side or part of your body, ensure you address the imbalances with corrective exercises designed by a Pilates instructor or qualified trainer. Tennis, squash, golf, or bowls are all examples that will result in an imbalanced physiology. This means you over-use or work more muscles than others. This creates imbalance in your neurophysiology and makes your body stronger in some areas and weaker in others. Left unchecked, this will present biomechanical imbalance that may result in muscle, nerve and skeletal degeneration and pain.

Pilates and Gyrokenesis® are excellent ways to rebalance and avoid injuries to reduce any downtime in these sports. These incredible movement modalities restore and support you to keep function, muscle mass and balance in your physical abilities as you age.

SHARON

How I keep fit and healthy

I am an avid horse rider, which requires using my legs and core to communicate with my horse and keep my balance while he moves. Caring for my horse involves lifting 20kg feed bags, using wheelbarrows to pick up manure, carrying the tack (bridles, saddle, stirrups, reins and so on) and other physical tasks like grooming, cleaning stables and washing out horse floats.

I share this with you to show you that there are many ways you can increase your incidental movement and build muscle without going to a gym or lifting weights. I call this being 'farm fit'. If horses are not your thing, get creative. What do you love to do that keeps you active and strong?

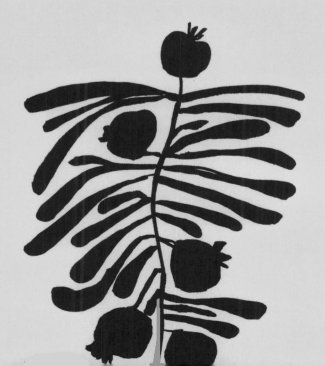

Stay calm.

As we embark
on Pillar Three...

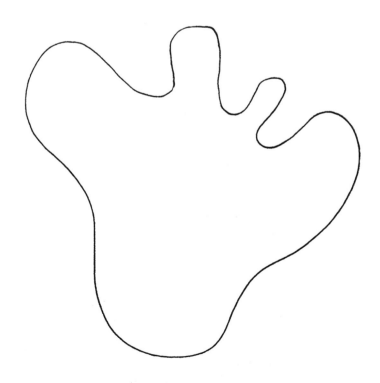

6.
EMOTIONAL
WELLBEING

Thoughts
could leave
deeper scars
than anything else.

MADAM POMFREY

THE HOGWARTS HEALER FROM HARRY POTTER

In this chapter, we peel back some of the layers of the human emotional landscape. We hope by the end of the chapter you will have a deeper understanding of how complex your inner world can be.

There can be a lot going on behind the 'window dressing' we show to the world. As you read through this chapter, it is important for you to note how you are feeling about the information you read and be kind to yourself. If you feel triggered by any of the following words, take some time to pause and reflect on the emotions that arise.

Have you ever noticed how any kind of pressure or stress becomes more of a struggle when you are emotionally upset? When our emotional selves are out of balance, we are less tolerant, our ability to complete tasks is compromised and we generally just want to crawl under a rock and escape from the world.

Your experience and the emotions that may arise as you read this chapter are unique to you, as you use your unconscious filters to navigate these emotional concepts. The intention of this chapter is to bring awareness to the hidden causes of emotional upheaval and provide some solutions. If you feel challenged whilst reading this chapter or feel emotionally confused or bruised, we encourage you to pause reading, take a deep breath and consider connecting with a mental health or emotional wellbeing counsellor. At the end of this book you will find a list of resources to support you.

What's your emotional IQ?

How often do you stop to think about the 'why' behind your emotions?

Having a good understanding of your emotional self and being able to *respond* to situations instead of *reacting* to them, is called emotional intelligence (EI). It can make the world of difference to the way in which you experience your life. Typically, we believe our feelings to be the result of some external influence, for example the way somebody else behaves, or something they say has affected the way we feel.

However, this isn't always true. For the most part, we don't tend to reflect on what might be driving us to feel a particular way about a situation; we tend to accept our emotions at their surface value.

If you can delve a little deeper, there is a rich opportunity to understand yourself. From there, you will be able to make deep and lasting change to your state of wellbeing and develop an increased capacity to cope with pressure and reduce stress.

ALEXITHYMIA

People with high levels of alexithymia (a condition best explored by a trained mental health specialist) have difficulty understanding and identifying their own emotions. They may suspect they are experiencing an emotion, but may not be able to name which emotion it is, or identify whether they are sad, angry or anxious. About 10 per cent of the population and about 50 per cent of people with autism have alexithymia.

For those on the spectrum, we could assume that autism somehow causes alexithymia, but it's worth remembering that you can have autism without alexithymia and vice versa. Although it is currently acknowledged that there are higher rates of alexithymia in people with autism, it's also noted that there are equally high rates in people with depression, eating disorders, schizophrenia, substance abuse as well as many other psychiatric and neurological conditions. If you have a diagnosed condition, it is best to review and discuss this chapter with your specialist.

THE MEANING BEHIND OUR BEHAVIOURS

Whether we realise it or not, deep down we all have fears that drive us to behave in certain ways - sometimes positively, sometimes not. Even if we know what a certain deep fear is, we tend to keep it to ourselves. We may share what upsets us or makes us angry, yet the underlying root cause of these feelings can go undetected and unnoticed for many years. Sadly, this often plays out in unconscious patterns of behaviour that we repeat over and over again. These are often best unravelled by a professional in human behaviour.

TALKING ABOUT YOUR FEELINGS

If you have someone in your life with whom you can divulge your deeper feelings, insecurities and worries, talking to them can help. A trusted friend or confidante can be a godsend. However, even the very best of friends (family or otherwise) may not be trained to ask the right questions that will allow you to truly pull apart the tapestry of your emotional self. Whether you have someone to confide in or not, it's best to consult with a qualified practitioner to unpack emotional wounds.

A QUESTION OF TRUST

It may be that you have trusted before, only to be exposed and let down. Unfortunately, this can result in a wall being built around your trust, where you now reside, confused about how you are actually feeling and not knowing what to do or where to turn. Maybe, in this state of sadness or depression that feels like it won't ever lift, you head to the doctor thinking there is something wrong with you: often their only solution is to offer medication.

A PLACE FOR MEDICINE?

Medication may be needed and can be helpful and, in some cases, is an essential tool for support. However, the blanket-prescription mentality to help patients deal with emotional upheaval does not always address the deeper issues. Potentially, prescription medicine can help you feel better for a while, but it doesn't teach you to regulate or understand your own emotions without the support of medication. Some of these medications have side effects which can create havoc with a person's health and cause further turmoil, so choosing to prescribe them needs careful consideration. Additionally, tempering feelings of sadness with medication levels out *all the emotions*, so it can impact your experience of joy and happiness as well. Asking your GP to refer you to a qualified mental health practitioner may be the best prescription, because they have more time to spend with and therefore listen to their patients and they are trained and qualified to view each case individually.

Health is the
greatest gift,
contentment
is the greatest
wealth, a trusted
friend is the
best relative,
a liberated mind
is the best bliss.

BUDDHA

HOW YOUR BELIEFS COLOUR YOUR WORLD

The feelings and thoughts you generate in response to every situation you are exposed to in your life creates a framework of beliefs that is stored deep in your subconscious. You are also influenced and imprinted by culture, society, parents, teachers, siblings, friends and the media (to name but a few), who teach you through words, imagery and their own actions and behaviours how you should process your experiences.

The way one person sees the world may be totally different to another person's view of it, depending on the filters created by their individual experiences. Because your perceptions of life and reality are filtered through your personal belief systems, what you think or perceive to *be* happening may be quite different to the truth of what *is* happening. We all have blind spots and limiting belief systems that colour our existence. By recognising and re-evaluating your inner world with a clear, unbiased perspective, you have the key to uncovering the story that can hinder your ability to feel and process the emotion.

YOUR SUBCONSCIOUS AND YOUR EMOTIONS

Your subconscious takes up about 90 per cent of your mind's capacity, and has a record-and-playback mechanism. It stores information that is invisible to your conscious mind and operates on autopilot. Every part of every day, your subconscious – your autopilot – responds or reacts to situations and events from both a physical and psychological stimulus.

This autopilot can also happen in day-to-day experiences at work or home. When you are busy and not paying attention to each moment, your subconscious mind can, and will, influence your behaviour based on your deeply embedded beliefs. Investigating our own beliefs is the key to unlocking our reactive behaviours and changing the way we feel about ourselves and the world. Why? Because some of the information stored in our subconscious may be distorted or untrue. This is usually because many of our foundational beliefs were created at a young age when our brain was still developing.

When we continue to make or reaffirm beliefs through adulthood, these decisions are usually influenced by earlier imprints. For example, let's say you overhear your parents saying that your conception was an unplanned accident. Whether it's shared verbally with you or not, being labelled 'the accident' will affect how you feel about yourself in relation to your family, how you feel about where and how you fit into the world and, even, perhaps, the direction you decide to take your life. Maybe you have always believed yourself to be 'different' and felt as though you didn't 'belong' or 'fit in' with the people in your life. But when you strip it back, does your conception being an 'accident' really matter to the people in your family? Being 'the accident' is only a bad thing if you believe it to be so.

WHY WE HAVE BELIEFS

Behind our beliefs is a drive to protect ourselves. When you experience situations in your life that you may find challenging, you tend to store information in your subconscious mind, in the form of beliefs. To protect yourself from any pain in the future you may form a belief that people cannot be trusted. This belief can stop you from sharing your vulnerabilities with people to avoid getting hurt again. However, at the same time, it can also stop you from connecting deeply with people – which may be something you really desire or need in your life.

Some beliefs are simple and some may be deeply embedded. Some of our beliefs are seen, such as having a deep faith in God or believing in equal rights for all of humanity. However, most are unseen and may be driving you to feel and behave in ways you often don't realise.

WHAT'S HOLDING YOU BACK?

Post-traumatic growth can come from lessons learnt through past trauma and difficult experiences. The tragedy is not what happened to you; this has already happened. The tragedy is the limiting negative belief about yourself that was put in play – relating to that event – that you still believe in – and continue to run with today.

What happened to you in the past may have been traumatic, and may have been a violation of your trust or your innocence. However, it is the negative belief that was created in response to the experience that is causing the damage and heartache today, preventing you from allowing your life to flourish. This is what will limit your full potential.

It is true that some events do change how we behave. However, you still have the potential to become someone who makes a wonderful contribution to yourself, your family, your wider community or the world. As difficult as it may sound, clearing past horrors, slights, rejections and hurtful behaviour so they do not define who you are today, is the way forward.

THE BRIGHT SIDE

You may have heard the saying 'every cloud has a silver lining'. How often do you take the time to reflect on the hidden good after experiencing a difficult situation?

The tendency to dwell on the negative and repeatedly replay the story of past hurts can keep you in emotional pain. Reframing your thoughts by seeking the positive lessons (no matter how small) assists you in your everyday recovery. Over time, the traumatic event will hold less power over your emotional life and can give you new skills that can help you and others.

CASE STUDY | DR KAREN

Regaining power after trauma

Over my career I have counselled many women who have experienced highly traumatic incidents of sexual assault, including child sexual abuse at the hands of family members. I vividly remember one such brave woman, Caroline, who disclosed for the first time the sexual abuse she endured at the age of 12 by an uncle. She had been too petrified of her mother's response to even consider disclosing the abuse, worried that she would be blamed.

Caroline brought up her fear that her two daughters, now school aged, may be exposed to the same trauma. She described being hypervigilant around any males who, in her mind, had the potential to perpetuate the abuse cycle with her daughters. She was worried that her mistrust of males may impact on her children's ability to form safe and trusting relationships with men in their future.

In that consultation we explored the question: What lessons can you take from that terrible trauma that can help your daughters now? She paused for a moment and said: 'I can teach my children to set boundaries about who can touch their bodies. I need them to know I have their back and will protect and believe them.'

I commented that she was as strong as a lioness protecting her cubs from danger, and her past trauma now provided her with the opportunity for her to have the conversation with her daughters that she was unable to have in her own childhood.

Caroline was able to 'find the good' from her trauma and move forward with a renewed confidence in her skills as a mother.

THE BLAME GAME

Often we use blame to deflect the pain of processing a certain emotion. Left unchecked, blaming can become a pattern of thinking, and even worse, a way of life. Blaming can keep you stuck in a continual cycle of blame, attack and defensive communication. Truly the only person who gets hurt in a blame cycle is you. You may find yourself striking out at those who want to help you, and all you're really doing is hurting yourself by jeopardising your relationships with others.

WHERE TO START

Identifying the maze of beliefs that colour our existence is something many prominent experts discuss. Psychotherapists speak of exposure therapy, which involves a client reappraising an event or a situation in life. Author and mind-body healing pioneer Brandon Bays speaks of allowing the body to release fears and emotions to connect with the truth. Author Byron Katie says to do 'The Work', a compassionate method of self-inquiry that can lead a person out of the victim maze and teaches us that we are not 'our story'.

Finding the right support is the best aid for moving through emotional pain. This could be through a deepening connection to your own spirituality, or working with a trained professional, who will ask you the right questions to unravel your beliefs. It's vitally important to understand that you are not defined by a 'story' that has happened to you.

If you are living with deep emotional fears or scars, tell someone, do something. In doing so, you will set yourself free to fully live again. Believe in yourself. Always keep hope in your heart as this can be the path to finding a better way to live. Countless women have done so, and you can, too.

Allow whatever comes to come. Allow whatever goes to go. Allow whatever stays to stay.

**PAPAJI
(H.W.L. POONJA)**

HOW EQUINE THERAPY CAN HELP

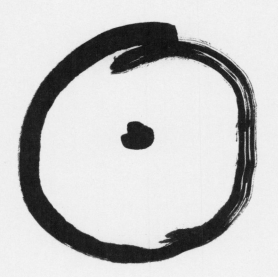

Sharon has had the pleasure of owning and being around horses all her life. She loves to share Equine Assisted Learning with people, using her horses. The focus during these sessions is on natural horsemanship, stress resilience, team building and leadership.

Equine therapy, or Equine Assisted/Facilitated Learning (EAL) (EFL) focuses on using the horse to bring to life human non-verbal communication, along with the power of breath and intention. Horses are finely tuned to humans and read every movement and facial expression. They also offer incredible insights to the facilitator about how the client is feeling and communicating. By reading the horse's body language, facilitators are able to share some powerful lessons in non-verbal communication and leadership between humans. This is usually most powerful when offered as a group learning, because the horse does not respond to each person the same way. These individual responses offer further insights to each participant. The facilitator is very skilled with horses and generally not qualified in any mental health modality as EAL is not delving into the mental or emotional state of the participants.

EAT (Equine Assisted Therapy) is offered by a qualified mental health or emotional wellbeing practitioner from various modalities such as psychiatry, Gestalt therapy, psychotherapy and counselling. This is usually offered one-on-one. During a session, the practitioner uses the herd of horses to bring to life unseen beliefs and behaviours by reading the interaction between the patient and the horses. This is a very powerful way to expose and heal emotional wounds and has been found to have an amazing impact on people with post-traumatic stress disorder (PTSD). Always check the qualifications of the practitioner in this modality. It is important that their credentials are valid and up to date.

THE RELATIONSHIP BETWEEN BELIEFS AND PRESSURE

Our ability to cope in any given situation depends upon how we feel and what we tell ourselves about it. For example, being called in to see the boss could induce panic: 'What have I done wrong?', or excited anticipation: 'Am I getting a promotion?'. Seeing a mouse in the kitchen could make you scream and jump on a chair, or conversely, you may calmly grab a broom to shoo it away. This is because our body's responses and reactions to the myriad pressures we face every day all stem from the unconscious mind – the way we are trained or imprinted to perceive the situation.

Our perception of a threat, real or imagined, can push us into the Red Zone (see Chapter 7: Stress and your nervous system). True stress management is an inwardly focused, ongoing awareness of how we see ourselves in relation to our external world. When you interrupt your usual response to a situation, you rewire your brain. Becoming more aware in each situation you find yourself in, and observing your usual reactions, you can then ask yourself if your perception of the situation is true and/or if it is life threatening. This way you can manage your life from the inside out, rather than trying to control the outside world.

Your ability to function with minimum reactions and calm curiosity in a busy technological world begins with open enquiry and inner reflection. The more you understand about how you think and feel in each moment, the more you can appreciate how your time-travelling mind can manipulate you into seeing something that does not exist (and may never have existed). When you are not being mindful, a figment of your fear can tell you a story of what *may* happen. You may then become anxious, stressed and/or panicky. This can then set off a host of physical reactions as a result of this stress-hormone response.

THE POWER OF BELIEF

Buried deep in your subconscious, a belief is a moment frozen in time. Each of us view our reality through the filter of our beliefs. Thoughts and feelings can come and go. Beliefs are hidden and frozen from the moment they come into being. Which means that sometimes we don't see what is truly in front of us, as our brain interprets what our eyes see through the filter of our beliefs.

Imagine an iceberg. The ice you see above the water is the conscious mind and is 10 per cent of our mind's capacity. Below the surface lives the other 90 per cent: your subconscious mind, which is filled with beliefs that rule your way of being. Both the conscious mind and the subconscious mind are often prisoners of 'seeing is believing'. According to some of the laws in quantum physics, stepping outside this cage offers us incredible potential in living the life we dream of living.

In medical research, the powerful influence of negative beliefs in shaping genetic expression and behaviour is called the 'nocebo effect'. This is a physical consequence of a belief that a certain substance or behaviour will cause harm. This is the opposite of a placebo - which may be an inert substance with no active ingredients given to an individual (while the individual believes it will do some good). It is estimated that pharmaceutical placebos 'work' 60 per cent of the time to deliver a positive outcome without the negative side effects of the real medication.

BELIEF HAS THE POWER TO KILL

The process of 'pointing the bone' (Kurdaitcha in indigenous language), was a well-established means of execution in the belief system of the Arrernte group of First Australians. The victim was usually a tribe member who had transgressed tribal law and had been condemned to death. The tribal elder acts as executioner by pointing a bone (made from kangaroo skeleton) at the accused who is then exiled to die. It is said these young men quickly perished because of their fixed belief in the Kurdaitcha system of justice. Similar stories are told in other indigenous cultures, including the practice of Voodoo in the Caribbean.

Why are we telling you this? Belief is a complete concept: you either believe or you don't. Beliefs have the power to unite us. However, they are also one of the major causes of division amongst humans. Our individual beliefs are coloured by our perception, shaped by our personality and are therefore not a universal truth. When we recognise that truths can co-exist simultaneously, we wake up to our own need to be right, which is often deeply embedded in our subconscious.

When we put our beliefs under the microscope we can begin to understand there are many layers. The deepest layers are often hidden from our own awareness. If belief is such an influencing factor in our health, how can we manage our belief structure? This is the juicy part. We can go deeply down the rabbit-hole or we can simply work on a different playing field.

DOWN THE RABBIT-HOLE

Becoming aware of your beliefs is crucial for personal growth. Beliefs begin to be imprinted into our subconscious from the moment we are born (some schools of thought believe it is from the moment of conception). Our environment shapes our belief structure; how our parents think and behave; how we interact with our siblings, teachers, friends and relatives; the economy of the house we grow up in; the schools we attend; the religion we are exposed to; the society and culture in which we grow up.

All these experiences affect how you interpret what happens to you, as well as impacting your self-esteem and world views, resulting in a belief structure deeply imbedded in your subconscious mind.

The subconscious mind is a bit like an operating system acting on autopilot. It records information and plays back the stored information to help you interpret the world and stay safe. It does not judge or evaluate what it records, it just documents it. The conscious mind is the part of the mind we are aware of: it thinks and plans, and is secretly, and constantly, affected by the subconscious mind. The conscious mind is a time traveller. It can skip from past to present to future, and does this every minute of every day, often unmanaged and unnoticed. This can be called a busy mind.

Delving into the unconscious mind to expose belief structures is the realm of The Journey workers, psychotherapists, Gestalt and holistic counsellors. A new emerging field called interpersonal neurobiology is investigating how the mind, brain and body interact to offer a perspective of ourselves and the world. It looks at what effect this has on the type of messages sent by the brain to tell our body how to respond.

WHAT IMPACT CAN YOUR THOUGHTS HAVE?

Our own thought process consistently and unconsciously embeds into our subconscious mind what we **don't** want to happen. The subconscious, your autopilot, that rules most of your behaviours, runs the usual script and you act accordingly.

For example: When we think 'I am fat', the subconscious mind records 'I am fat'. Our beliefs then ensure that the body retains fat. When we think: 'I want more love in my life', the subconscious records this message of wanting more love, so that we experience wanting more love. When we think, 'I am getting a cold', our subconscious records us actually getting a cold. When we say, 'I am overwhelmed and stressed', this is what plays out in real life.

THE CONSCIOUS AND SUBCONSCIOUS MIND

Your conscious mind and subconscious mind are imprisoned within your own structured belief system. Let's look: when you are born you are pure, innocent and full of potential. As a child you saw the world through your imagination. (Sadly, parents, teachers and the world around us limit our imagination to what is real. This can limit your ability to manifest whatever you may feel you are lacking in your life.)

The wonder of your imagination is that there are no limits, there's no need to distinguish between what's 'real' and what's 'not real'. This means that you can bring to 'life' the existence (or fruition of goals or love, etc) you've always wanted or desired for yourself. This is what we call 'manifesting'.

THE WONDERS OF MANIFESTING

There's only one rule when it comes to manifesting the life you've always wanted: there are no rules. Throw the rule book out the window and let your imagination run free. Don't worry about the 'how' or the potential hurdles; simply think 'what if anything was possible'. What would that world look like for you?

By choosing to challenge the status quo, you can act to shift thoughts and perspectives to marry with what you want to happen. The 30-day helpful thought and action challenge on the following pages can help you begin your journey. Each day you'll see that we have suggested a change in the language many people typically use, in order to help you change your focus or emotions surrounding a situation.

Take notes to help you be aware if there is a shift in your perception, during, or by the end of the challenge.

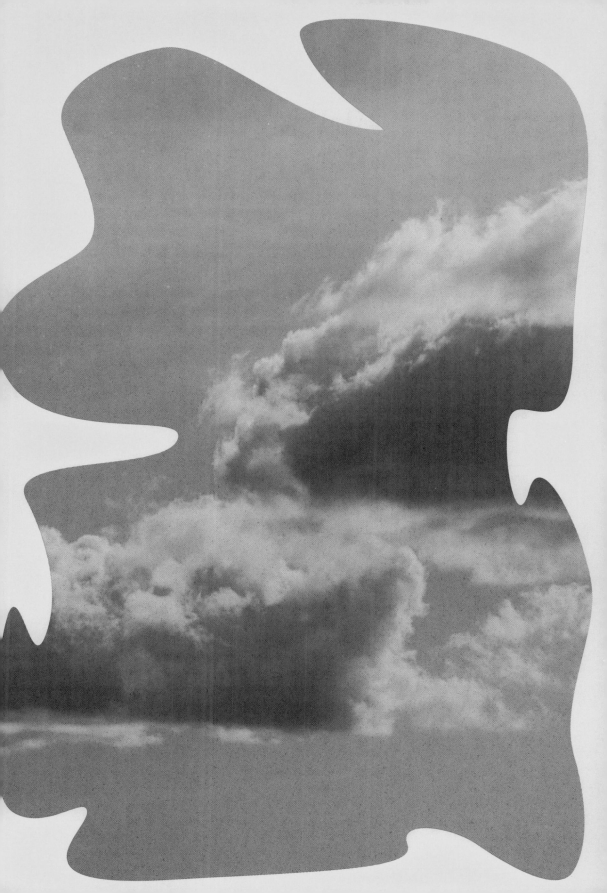

YOUR 30-DAY HELPFUL THOUGHT AND ACTION CHALLENGE

DAY 1

'I will drink at least 2 litres of filtered water today because my body needs to be hydrated.'

DAY 2

'I will make time to walk in nature today to move and clear my mind.'

DAY 3

'I am sleeping better every night, and this will allow my body to rest and repair.'

DAY 4

'I have the time to prepare a balanced evening meal, because nourishing myself is self-care.'

DAY 5

'Today I will choose extra movement, this will help me to enjoy life more and live well.'

DAY 6

'Today I will find time to put my feet up, because 'me-time' is important for my health and wellbeing.'

DAY 7

'I love eating nourishing foods because I feel good after eating them. My body has all the ingredients it needs to do its healing and recovery job.'

DAY 8

'I worked hard in my exercise session today. I know this is improving my strength and fitness which will add to my feeling good about the care I take of myself.'

DAY 9

'I enjoy quiet time alone. I deserve to create many of these moments in my life, because my body needs time to rest and recover.'

DAY 10

'I feel grateful to be able to prepare a nourishing meal for myself, my family and friends. It's how I share my care and love for myself and others.'

DAY 11

'I will choose the stairs today, to take every opportunity to get extra movement in my day and build strong muscles in my legs.'

DAY 12

'I look forward to strategic rest, taking time to relax and the space to be creative for my mental, emotional and physical wellbeing.'

DAY 13

'I love eating different vegetables because they keep my gut bugs happy – when they are happy, I am happy.'

DAY 14

'I choose to exercise because I get stronger and fitter. This makes me feel alive.'

DAY 15

'I pay attention to slowing down my breathing during the day to calm my nervous system and keep myself regulated.'

DAY 16

'Chewing my food well is helping me to improve my digestion. This helps me to absorb essential nutrients from the food.'

DAY 17

'I will enjoy challenging my body today because I feel like I have achieved something: I get fitter and stronger. It's a win-win.'

DAY 18

'Being present is joyful because I open my senses and notice what is in the moment right now: a butterfly, a gorgeous smell, a loved one, or even a perfect blue sky.'

DAY 19

'Fresh food is delicious and my body converts it to give me energy.'

DAY 20

'I can do some form of movement or exercise today because I take care of myself.'

DAY 21

'I am truly grateful for simple things in my life; a kind word, a smile, having some food and having connection with the local community.'

DAY 22

'I am happy with 'me' today: I am enough. I enjoy incorporating healthy food into my daily eating plan.'

DAY 23

'Living each day as it comes allows me to meet every day with positivity and open curiosity for what may happen.'

DAY 24

'I respect my body's needs and do my very best to support and nurture my body and myself.'

DAY 25

'I am more than a work in progress. I am an incredible living, breathing being and each day is joyous.'

DAY 26

'I love to hear my heart beat faster and my breath increase when I exercise. It makes me feel strong and healthy.'

DAY 27

'I choose to live in the moment, to explore each day as a brand-new one, full of possibilities.'

DAY 28

'I no longer weigh myself. I choose to eat well, move well and think helpful thoughts.'

DAY 29

'I choose to move as much as possible today – in many and various ways – because I know the benefits of regular movement.'

DAY 30

'I love my life. It is a life that I have created just for me. I am now able to share my joy for life with others.'

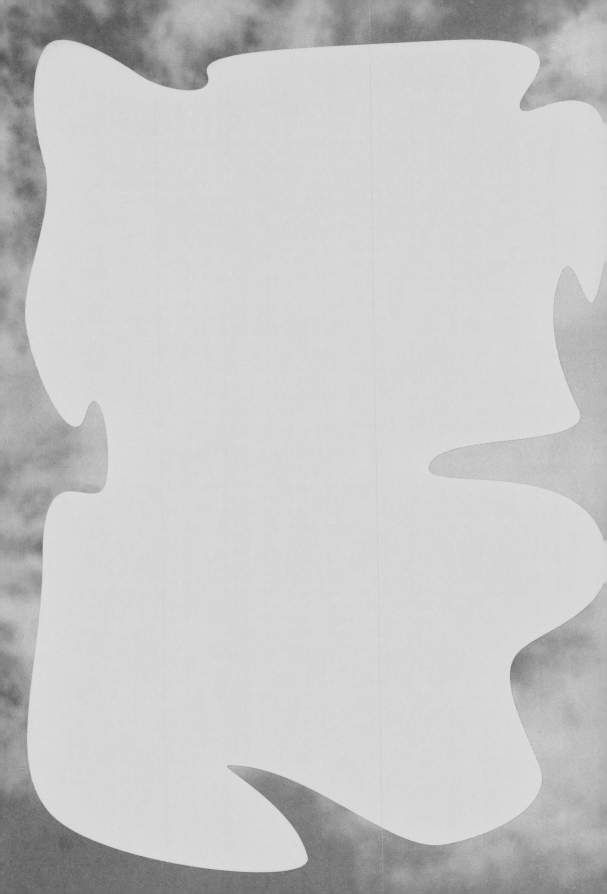

Imagination is
more important
than knowledge.
For knowledge
is limited,
whereas imagination
embraces the
entire world,
stimulating progress,
giving birth
to evolution.

ALBERT EINSTEIN

THE POWER OF MEDITATION

HUGH JACKMAN

on

Transcendental Meditation

Sharon asked her friend Hugh Jackman, star of the
Wolverine X-Men film series and *The Greatest Showman*
(amongst others), and one of Australia's favourite actors,
how a daily ritual of transcendental meditation has helped
him achieve his goals.

'It's been twenty-two years since I started meditating. I've pretty much always done it at least once a day and a lot of the time it's twice a day. I would say starting meditation was a massive turning point in my life. I was in my mid-twenties when I started, and up until that point I'd been very reactive to much of what happened in my life. I was a searcher for meaning, but meditation gave me a deeper understanding of who I was, why we were here, what life was about. It somehow anchored everything I did, gave it a context where not every single activity in my life was the be all and end all; that there was some foundation underneath it that felt like home, or the "real" me. I wasn't so dependent on success or failure, on any given thing on any given day, but rather there was a sense of myself beyond good or bad, success or failure, and that was revealed to me through meditation.

'Finding that peace, that stillness within, a sense of calm and bliss, started to naturally appear. I wouldn't say it was immediate. It did take a while, but that's what started to appear and it has given me a kind of perspective which I've been so grateful for as my life has gone on.

'On a very practical level, I find it is the purest form of revitalising myself that I know of, even more than sleep. After meditating I have a finer energy than before - it's the equivalent of pulling back a bow on a bow and arrow. I find that once I've meditated, any activity I tackle afterwards, for a fair amount of time, is much clearer, more succinct and direct, and more productive than it would be otherwise. Sometimes I'll just fall asleep! I really trust now that whatever happened in meditation is exactly what I need. Sometimes it takes me a while for my mind to settle down, sometimes ideas will pop up during meditation - creative ideas or solutions to problems - that I probably never would have discovered if I'd sat down and tried to solve it with a pen and paper, weighing up pros and cons.

'It also has brought me closer to people. The process of meditation not only brings me closer to the true version of myself, but it makes it easier for me to really see other people around me and to connect with them.

'In terms of the ritual of it, I'm aware that it's hard for a lot of people to commit, and it has been hard for me at times, sometimes I've had to push through. It is a form of discipline, but I do believe that the goal of tapping into that natural bliss, the natural consciousness and truth that is within us all that meditation is the key for, does require some work, some discipline.

'Meditation is all about doing nothing, and ironically, sometimes it can seem quite hard to do that. We're so addicted to achieving and doing and thinking, and we almost enjoy the adrenaline. So to just switch off can be difficult. I wouldn't say it's completely concrete for me, doing it twice a day, but it's 80 or 90 per cent concrete. But as it's gone on, it's become more of a joy and less of a duty, and the benefits have certainly been astonishing for me.

'I find that I can now recognise someone else who meditates quite easily. There is something about them, a sense of alertness and detachment from the machinations of daily life, and a sense of joy and of bliss. They are calm and very easy to be around.

'The beauty of meditation, for me is that you do not need any skill. You don't need any faith; you don't need to believe in it. It's just a technique – you just have to show up. Whether you believe in it or not doesn't matter, the benefits will be there for everybody. And it's literally everybody – there's not a person on the planet who can't meditate. I hear people say, 'I'm not the type of person for it' or 'I can't sit still', but that's just not true. I know many people who do it who seem like the opposite person for meditation. It doesn't matter what religion you are, what race you are, none of it matters. I see it totally benefiting everybody.'

WHY MEDITATION IS A MUST

Meditation is the process of allowing yourself to become still, to observe your thoughts without judgement. With practice you will find space between your thoughts: with this comes peace and contentment. Finding time to meditate helps you recruit your CEO brain. This part of your brain is your best friend when you are regulating your brain activity and observing your daily life (find out more about your CEO brain in Chapter 7 and 8).

There are many different styles of meditation. Find a style that suits you - you may like to join a meditation group or choose an app to assist you on this journey.

When you first begin your meditation practice, start slowly and approach it with curiosity, rather than expectation. It can be a good idea to set aside 10 minutes of your day to focus on your inner world and build from there as you become more patient with your practice. As time goes on, notice if your practice is helping you regulate your mood, energy and emotions for the rest of your day.

The first thing you may notice is how busy your mind is, and how many thoughts are racing through each moment. This is the beginning. Simply sit, watch and breathe. Your practice will become natural to you, just you, observing your mind, without attaching to any thought.

YOUR RELATIONSHIP WITH YOURSELF

No matter who we are, what we own, how we live, what we do for work, family or no family, we all have an inner world hidden from external view. Here lies the relationship you have with yourself. This relationship you have with yourself is the most important relationship in your life, as it impacts every aspect of your being, both internally and externally. We believe that no matter your current State of Being, adapting and learning more about your inner world is key to a healthy life.

Some of the solutions on the following pages may be normal for you and some may be a new way to perceive your inner and outer world.

1.
The importance of love and connection

Sharon says:

'In 2014, I attended a three-day seminar led by Dr. Deepak Chopra (author, leader in meditation and alternative medicine advocate). An audience member asked him to explain how we are all connected or "one". Without skipping a beat, Deepak told us to look at the fans in the room. Then to look at the lights, air conditioner and speakers. He explained that each [of these items] expressed themselves independently, in a way that is needed for their function; yet they were each connected to something that gave them power – electricity. All electricity comes from the same source. Without that electrical source none of those devices would be able to function.

'According to the principles of quantum physics, at the deepest level of existence we are all a part of the whole universe – existing from the same source of energy.

'Emotionally, everyone needs two things in life. The first is to be accepted and understood, to have a voice, which, when used, is truly heard by the people, friends and family you love and admire.

'The second is love. You will have seen first-hand proof that regardless of position, power, celebrity or economic status, being loved and loving others is what is truly valuable in life. It is the very essence of what it means to be human, yet we meet so many people who are disconnected and full of fear about life. Some people don't even realise how detached they have become from themselves, from each other, and the planet.'

FACT
Loneliness is likely to increase your risk of death by 26 per cent.

2.
The power of giving

Sharon says:

'I was introduced to the wonderful Stephen G. Post through a mutual friend. Stephen is a Professor of Preventive Medicine and Founding Director of the Center for Medical Humanities, Compassionate Care and Bioethics at Stony Brook University School in the United States. He is an author, published researcher, and President of The Institute for Research on Unlimited Love.

'In my interview with Dr Post, he explained that there is substantial research that connects doing good with living a longer, healthier, happier life. He believes that forgiveness, altruism, compassion and service are vital for longevity and a healthy heart. He also told me – with a glint in his eye – that he truly believes that love (not the romantic, humankind) is the ultimate power that created the universe. He likens love to gravity.

'On a more worldly level, Stephen talked about the powerful research on the act of giving. Not in giving material things such as money, but giving as an action that shows another person you care. This might be listening, volunteering your assistance, smiling at others and spending quality time with loved ones. Giving is also receiving, as you are then allowing another person the pleasure of giving. When we really give from our heart and soul, the benefit is twofold. There is the pleasure we feel when we are moved by our own actions and the biochemical release to our cells that enhances our body's healing capabilities.

'That day, Stephen did nothing but "give" to me; he was walking his talk. His strong message to all of us is: "The act of giving makes us more resilient and healthier and that research shows it is very helpful to assist in the prevention of many chronic diseases".'

We believe in the power of giving: give to yourself, to others. Give freely, without expectations, baggage or resentment.

Here's something to practise: the next time you volunteer your time (whether it's at your child's school, helping a friend out or at a community event), check in with yourself. Do you feel resentful for giving up your time? Are you giving your time and energy so that you are recognised and thanked? There's nothing wrong with feeling this way, but it can take away from the unconditional act of giving. It may be that you need to check your boundaries are in place before you give. For instance, instead of volunteering your entire Saturday morning to help at a local event, put some boundaries into place such as: 'I can give you two hours of my time on Saturday to help.' By being precise in what you can give and offer there's little room for confusion (or for people taking advantage of your good nature!).

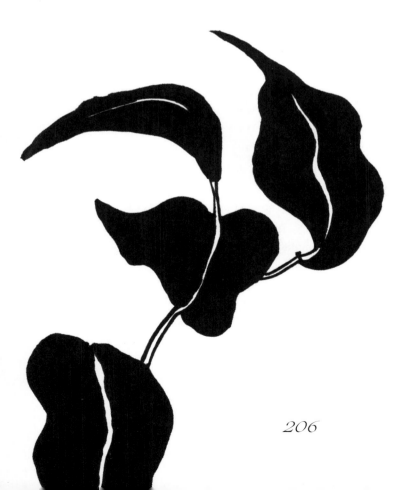

STEPHEN G POST,
PROFESSOR OF PREVENTIVE MEDICINE

FORGIVENESS AS MEDICINE

Forgiveness reduces the powerful mixture of anger, hatred and fear that comes with seeing ourselves as victims. Chronic anger has been well documented to have harmful effects on the cardiovascular and immune systems. People who score high on forgiveness are less likely to be depressed, anxious, hostile, narcissistic or exploitative and are less likely to become dependent on drugs and nicotine.

Combat veterans suffering from PTSD experience less depression and fewer symptoms of trauma if they are able to forgive themselves and others. High forgivers show less reactivity in blood pressure and arterial stiffness. In contrast, those who score low in forgiveness show higher blood pressure and slower recovery.

THE EXPERTS' VIEW ON FORGIVENESS

Cardiologist and physician Dr. Jason Kaplan and cardiologist Dr. Ross Walker, refer to themselves as 'integrative cardiologists'. These brilliant and innovative men are changing the way we consider and manage heart disease (at time of writing, the number one killer of Australians and many people in Western countries). They both believe love and connection is a major factor in the formula to reverse and prevent heart disease and stroke. In fact, Dr Walker says that love and connection are the best 'drugs' he can offer his patients.

STEPS TOWARDS FORGIVENESS

So, how do you learn to forgive? The pathway to forgiveness is through empathy. By considering the situation from the perspective of someone who you believe has hurt you, you may be able to recognise that they are not only a perpetrator, but they are also someone who has been hurt through life themselves. Or they have no idea that they wounded you through their inability to stay out of their Red Zone (see Chapter 7). Forgiveness gives you the control to move on. Sometimes we need to forgive, not for the other person but simply in order to set ourselves free.

FORGIVE AND FEEL BETTER

- Forgiving others improves health more than being forgiven
- Forgiveness alleviates depression
- Forgiveness boosts mood and reduces anger
- Forgiveness lowers stress hormones
- Forgiveness preserves close relationships

STEP ONE

Forgive yourself first

It is said that we find it harder to forgive ourselves than others because we are so self-critical. We all bear emotional scars and work tirelessly to hide our deepest fears, because we're scared of being exposed and being found vulnerable. Yet vulnerability, according to international best-selling author Brené Brown, allows us to change our lives and become 'wholehearted people'. There's usually a bit of anger in the mix, too – for something we should have done, or not done. How can we forgive anyone else if we cannot forgive ourselves? Forgiveness is central to thriving in life. If you are challenged by forgiving yourself and/or others and need support to move what's holding you back, it could be time to seek professional help and support. Find a therapist, get to the bottom of your deepest fears, forgive yourself and live, really live, your life.

Our **Resources** section is a great place to help you find a therapist to help guide you on your journey.

STEP TWO

Teach forgiveness to the young

As we age and our values shift, we become more forgiving. Research shows that young children are the least willing to forgive and that younger adults need to be encouraged to forgive. One study found that children who imagined 'getting back' at friends in imaginary scenarios had fewer best friends and were less accepted by their peers.

We gain our sense of self at an early age. Any emotional wound experienced in early childhood has a lasting effect on our self-esteem, our ability to see truth and how we see the world.

Paul Connolly, Professor at Queen's University Belfast, is internationally recognised for his research on early childhood. In 2002, a study was conducted of 352 children from across Northern Ireland aged from three to six. These children came from either a Roman Catholic or Protestant upbringing and through the influence of their families, local communities and schools, the children had already learned to loathe and fear one another, deeply absorbing hatred and prejudice by age five.

Children learn what they live. Wouldn't it be better to expose them to the power of forgiveness, rather than setting them on a path to continue a fight long after you are gone? Everyone has an opportunity to inspire the next generation to be more compassionate and understanding of other people.

STEP THREE

Learn the limits of a grudge

From an evolutionary perspective, it is a natural reaction to become angry when somebody has hurt you; it's a form of self-protection. According to Kenneth Pargament, a Spiritually Integrated Psychotherapist and author, anger, fear, hurt and resentment are actually coping techniques that help us stay in touch with our energy and power to help us survive. His research shows that hurt is actually a source of comfort. It reminds us that we deserve better. What's more, expressing resentment can help remind others of our difficulties.

However, according to this author and psychotherapist, there is a fine line between feeling hurt and allowing hurt to rule our life. When you get trapped in a cycle of hatred and bitterness it is simply then hurting yourself.

STEP FOUR

How to let go of a grudge

Kenneth suggests practicing a metaphysical exercise: 'Imagine taking a permanent marker and writing "grudge" on your palm. Let the ink dry, then try to wash it off with soap and water. Little by little it will become lighter with every wash. Forgiveness is a process. With practice, your burden becomes lighter every day and your body becomes a better healer of itself.'

STEP FIVE

The power of an apology

Julie Exline is a Professor of Psychology with a special interest in the virtues of humanity and forgiveness. She found that a sincere apology helps to restore a relationship and wash away resentment and bitterness: 'A powerful apology is admitting responsibility for a mistake, expressing remorse and offering to repair the situation'.

According to Stephen G. Post, research shows that true remorse conveys distress, self-awareness and regret. It also elicits empathy from the person who has been hurt. His advice is to always apologise from the heart, with absolute sincerity.

If you are waiting for an apology from someone and it is not coming, try to have compassion and empathy for them. They may be suffering because they are unable to forgive themselves and, as a result, are unable to apologise to you. They may not know how to apologise, or may believe it's a weakness to do so. Not apologising can often show up their weakness, or expose their fear of failure. Remember, waiting in resentment for an apology that may never come is only hurting you, not them.

STEP SIX

Be the change you wish to see in the world

There are many examples of 'being the change you wish to see in the world', a phrase commonly associated with the humanitarian Gandhi. Think of volunteers the world over, helping the homeless or disadvantaged, offering their assistance to deal with natural disasters, raising money for various causes and so on, all of them with no expectation of recompense. What can you do today that allows you to contribute to the greater good of humanity? As the now well-known expression promotes: 'pay it forward'.

STEP SEVEN

Nature does nurture

Another positive contribution to connection and health is our very real need to regularly be in nature. A 2018 study showed that the awe we feel in nature may help lower levels of inflammatory proteins, which improves our health and wellness.

According to the study, whenever we experience awe in the presence of nature, art and spirituality, we get a boost to our body's immune defence system. Positive emotions are associated with lower levels of inflammatory cytokines, which are proteins that signal the immune system to work harder. Sustained higher levels of cytokines are associated with poor health and chronic diseases such as Type 2 diabetes, heart disease, arthritis, dementia and clinical depression.

We all need to find our flow with, and within, nature. Maybe, for you, it's a walk in the park every day, a swim in the ocean, planting some food or flowers and spending time with your pets. The human species is designed to connect with the elements of Mother Nature. When you rise with the sun and go to bed early, your body flows into its natural circadian rhythm. It is this rhythm that is the foundation for your wellbeing. This essential rhythm is kept in check by your connection to yourself, to one another, and to Mother Nature.

For more information about how Mother Nature recharges your body, read about Qi in Chapter 8.

STEP EIGHT

Boundaries

Boundaries are safe environments – whether it's physical, emotional or spiritual – we create in order to help ourselves thrive. Personal boundaries are where our internal world meets the external world, and how we preserve our sense of self and wellbeing. By considering where and what your boundaries are, you communicate to yourself and others what you will, and won't, accept. Boundaries are indicative of the way we treat ourselves and how we would like others to treat us: personally and professionally.

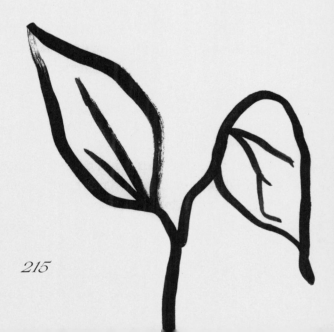

CASE STUDY | SHARON

Learning about consistency and boundaries

As a horse rider, I am interested in learning new and meaningful ways to communicate with my horses. Just like humans, horses have defined personalities and styles of communication so, interestingly, what we learn about interacting with horses can parallel the way we interact with humans. I have spent many years working with horse trainer John Wicks (John is a multiple Australian Reining Champion) and have learnt much horse sense from this unassuming cowboy.

One of the most important things John taught me, in fact, was about setting boundaries. 'That horse will do whatever you accept,' he said to me one day during a gruelling riding lesson. 'Horses need good leadership; your horse does not understand grey, he sees things in black and white; it is either wrong or right. If you are inconsistent with what you accept from him, you are not being fair to him. He needs you to be clear and consistent.' Long after the lesson I was thinking about boundaries and communication in general, and I realised that John's advice could be applied to many parts of life.

HOW TO MAINTAIN CLEAR AND CONSISTENT BOUNDARIES

In order to look after our health and be successful in whatever roles we fill in our lives (such as parent, employee, partner or manager), we need to maintain clear and consistent boundaries. Danielle Di-Masi, communication specialist, has a great analogy about the importance of boundaries. She uses airlines as an example.

We are all aware of the airline boundaries. As passengers, we know we need to be at the gate by a certain time, that we need to sit in our designated seat and that there are limitations to our luggage allowances. We accept these and many more rules because the airline boundaries are clearly communicated and are consistently enforced. Imagine if we turned up late, with too much luggage, wanting to sit anywhere because we had not been told otherwise. We would not be allowed on the plane. Aside from becoming confused and upset, we would argue that these rules should be communicated clearly.

It works much the same way in your everyday life. We need to understand our own boundaries – what we are comfortable with and what we are not – and communicate this to the people in our lives, so that they know what acceptable behaviour is. Imagine how confusing it would be for your workmates if one day it is fine for them to tease you about something because you are in a good mood or feeling good about yourself, but the next day your mood changes and, in response to their teasing, you become upset. They would likely become defensive and confused and it may change how they interact with you in the future.

Let's look at another example. Children are the ultimate boundary testers and they need firm and consistent boundaries in order to understand what's okay and what isn't. Imagine that one day it is okay for your children to behave a certain way and the next day, because you are tired, you yell at them for the same or similar behaviour. When we change our mind about what's okay and what's not in response to our emotional state it is confusing for both adults and children.

This can be a factor in why relationships and communication begin to break down. People in our life need to know and respect where our boundaries are. However, we have the responsibility to be clear about where and what they are. We need to remain consistent and reinforce our boundaries when they get transgressed. Communicate in a kind, respectful voice. Be clear about setting your boundaries and be consistent in monitoring and communicating respectfully when your boundaries are dented or crushed.

SETTING PERSONAL HEALTHY LIFESTYLE BOUNDARIES

Healthy boundaries are a crucial component of self-care. Why? Whether it's at work or in our personal relationships, poor boundaries can lead to resentment, anger and burnout.

To get into, and stay in a **Thriving State of Being**, it's important to know the difference between what you want, and what your body needs. You then need to set clear boundaries to support healthy outcomes.

You may *want* to indulge in eating sugary food, regularly drink as much alcohol as you wish, party hard every weekend and not do enough exercise, all while hoping it doesn't impact on your health.

However, we all know that this isn't how our body (or anybody's body!) works. There are consequences to your actions. When you moderate 'what you want' with more of 'what you need' by setting some personal care boundaries, your health will usually become a closer match to what it is you desire. This may be, for you, a life that's as functional as possible, full of happiness and contentment. This doesn't mean a dull and strict life;

life should not be about rules, it needs to be fluid. Above all, it should be enjoyed, in a healthy, positive way.

IT'S ALL ABOUT PROPORTIONS

This is where we'd like to remind you about the 80:20 lifestyle guide we spoke about in Chapter 3. Let's expand on the theme here. Eighty per cent of the time you will do what you *need* to do to support your body, mind and spirit to be healthy. The remaining 20 per cent of the time you can live a little (without blowing all your good habits completely out of the water).

If you feel out of balance, it's generally because you have not been clear with yourself about your personal boundaries. It's like the parent has gone out and left the kid at home without any rules, so they over-eat, drink too much and party/work all night! Except now you are your own parent. Unless you supervise yourself, no one else is likely to do it for you (even if they do, you will probably resent them for trying to control your life).

By setting healthy lifestyle boundaries you can avoid the internal debate you may face when you want something, even though you know it could eventually hurt you. For example, if your chosen boundary is to not drink alcohol from Monday to Thursday, and you bleed this boundary by having 'just the one on Wednesday night', you may have feelings of remorse and guilt. This can lead to an unnecessary cycle of self-bullying. Avoid arguing and debating the point in your mind: stay firm and introduce some healthy distractions, such as enjoying a long, hot bath or calling a friend. And always remind yourself that maintaining your own boundaries is for your own benefit, both long- and short-term.

That said, when you're creating your boundaries, remember to leave some leeway. Feeling deprived is not the way to sustain good habits.

Remember, *it is what you do most of the time that will have the most impact on your healthy life.*

SIGNS OF UNHEALTHY BOUNDARIES	SIGNS OF HEALTHY BOUNDARIES
Trusting no one – trusting anyone	Determining what is a safe boundary for relationships of all kinds
Not noticing when someone else displays inappropriate boundaries	Remain centred within your boundaries and notice when any breach happens and respectfully remind others what feels safe and OK for you
Talking at an intimate level within the first few meetings	Honouring your own personal values despite what others want
Feeling obliged to permit another person's sexual desires	Saying no until you feel comfortable and safe
Going against your personal values or rights to please another person	Revealing a little of yourself at a time, then checking to see how the other person responds to your sharing
Falling in love with someone who reaches out because you just want to be needed and loved	Keeping a safe distance physically and emotionally to allow time for you to find out if there is true compatibility
Falling in love too quickly	Showing interest yet taking your time to decide whether a potential relationship will be good for you
Being overwhelmed by a person – preoccupied	Trusting your own decisions
Touching a person or being touched without consent	Asking a person or being asked by a person before touching
Taking as much as you can get for the sake of getting	Defining your truth, as you see it
Giving as much as you can give for the sake of giving	Knowing you are worthy, you also have needs which should be noticed by those closest to you
Letting others define you	Being who you are, authentic and wise
Letting others direct your life	Talking to yourself with gentleness, humour, love and respect, live the life you desire
Allowing someone to take as much as they can from you	It is your responsibility to communicate your wants, needs and desires

'NO' IS A COMPLETE SENTENCE

Setting boundaries can take some time and practise. The more you practise being firm and truthful about your own wants and needs, the easier it will become to live a life within your own truth and comfortable boundaries. Here are some examples to help you start setting your boundaries as the situation arises.

When you say 'No' to others, you say 'Yes' to yourself.

INSTEAD OF...	TRY...
Saying 'yes' to an invite for something you don't want to attend	'I really appreciate you inviting me, sadly I won't be able to make it this time'
'I'd like to, but I'm really tired and I'm really busy, but it sounds good'	'So sorry, I just can't make it this time'
'Let me check my diary.' [But you have no intention of doing so!]	'Thank you for thinking of me, sadly I am really time poor right now and can't help sorry'
'Sure, maybe'	'Sorry It doesn't work for me at the moment'
'Sure I can do that work after I've finished this project'	'This project may not be for me, it sounds really exciting though, hope it goes well for you'
'Of course I'll come rock-climbing/ballet/jogging/weightlifting with you'	'Um, sorry that's not my thing. I can't wait to hear how you enjoy it'
Answering work calls/emails at any time of the day or night	'Thank you for connecting with me, I set one/three hours a day to answer emails and will get back to you as soon as I can'

HOW TO SET YOUR 80:20 BOUNDARIES – SOME EXAMPLES

The following examples of personal health boundaries may help you to understand if you're new to the game. You might want to implement a couple at a time and incrementally build up, so that the shift feels more manageable.

PERSONAL HEALTH BOUNDARIES – 80 PER CENT OF YOUR TIME

- ✓ I need seven to eight hours of sleep every night
- ✓ I need to be in bed before 10pm
- ✓ I do not eat fast or processed foods
- ✓ The majority of my diet will be certified organic
- ✓ I will only buy humanely raised, free-range, biodynamic or organically reared meats or I choose for humane reasons to exclude eating all meats and fish
- ✓ I will reduce/eliminate gluten and/or dairy from my diet
- ✓ I will prepare and eat healthy meals to nourish myself and my family
- ✓ I need a minimum of four alcohol-free nights per week and a minimum of one alcohol-free month per year.
- ✓ I need to drink two litres of still water every day
- ✓ I will not drink soft drinks
- ✓ I will have one (never more than two) caffeinated drink, such as tea or coffee, a day and drink it before midday
- ✓ I will commit to an exercise program

✓ I will meditate, do Qi Gong or practise visualisations every second day

✓ I will be firm in my boundaries within my relationships (i.e. the way they speak to me or treat me)

✓ I will only develop relationships with people I trust and respect

✓ I will recycle

✓ I will connect with nature every day

✓ I will continue to work in the same job only if I love what I do

✓ I will not allow my work to rule my life, yet I will give my all while I am at work

✓ I will ask for help when I need it

✓ I will prioritise spending time in my Blue Zone (find out more in Chapters 7 and 8)

Once you have identified your priority list to support you, or keep you in a **Thriving State of Being**, you can then begin to implement these statements in a way that suits you.

PERSONAL HEALTH BOUNDARIES – 20 PER CENT OF YOUR TIME

✓ I can eat good-quality 70 per cent dark chocolate

✓ I choose to eat certified organic corn chips/potato chips

✓ I can enjoy sparkling water

✓ I can enjoy good-quality red wine and/or white wine as well as mixer drinks

✓ I can eat a good-quality dessert

✓ I can lie on the couch watching television or go to the cinema

✓ I can eat out at restaurants

✓ I can eat healthy, hand-made, sustainably produced burgers or other higher quality takeaway foods

It does not matter what your personal health boundaries are, as long as they match your intended outcome. For example, if you want to lose body fat, it does not make sense to drink alcohol or eat chocolate every day. It does, however, make sense to eat healthy, organic balanced meals, get regular sleep and exercise. It also gives you freedom – even if you want to lose body fat – to enjoy a glass of red wine and organic dark chocolate on a Friday night, while watching your favourite TV show. Rather than seeing your positive health behaviours as rewarding your efforts, think about and focus on balancing your health goals with your lifestyle.

Be honest about what you want to achieve. Then consolidate it by setting boundaries you can honestly and consistently live by. Remember, you only need willpower at the start. You may want to engage a friend or coach to keep you motivated while the positive benefits of the change are being cemented. The very act of doing something regularly creates the habit and wires it into your brain as being normal.

You may need to adjust your boundaries occasionally, depending on your state of health.

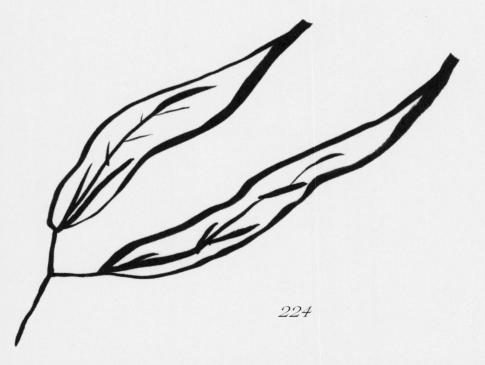

It's your turn!

WHAT ARE YOUR HEALTHY BOUNDARIES
(FOR 80 PER CENT OF THE TIME)?

Answer the following questions to help get you started on your boundary-building journey. Ask yourself these questions honestly while considering what you need to do in order to truly thrive. Write down your answers on a separate sheet of paper. You may wish to refer back to your answers as you continue on your journey towards stronger boundaries.

- How many hours of sleep each night do I need?

- How many alcohol-free nights a week do I need?

- Which foods do I need to eat most of the time?

- Which foods do I need to avoid?

- How much incidental movement do I need to do each day?

- How many exercise sessions do I need to do each week?

- What will I never do in my 80 per cent?

- What boundaries will I use for my 20 per cent?

- What do I enjoy that will not compromise my health goals?

- What is still off limits?

- What do I need to allow myself to have/do/experience without feeling guilty?

The Guest House

This being human is a guest house.

Every morning a new arrival.

A joy, a depression, a meanness, some momentary
awareness comes as an unexpected visitor.

Welcome and entertain them all!

Even if they are a crowd of sorrows, who violently sweep
your house empty of its furniture.

Still, treat each guest honourably.

They may be clearing you out for some new delight.

The dark thought, the shame, the malice, meet them at the
door laughing, and invite them in.

Be grateful for whoever comes, because each has been sent
as a guide from beyond.

RUMI

SUGGESTIONS AND SOLUTIONS

Healthy boundary setting in your present state

DEPLETED STATE OF BEING

In a depleted state you may need to adjust the percentage to 90:10 or even 100 per cent while your body requires more support to re-establish equilibrium and heal. Spending time resting and relaxing is essential and should be a major priority for you. Read the boundaries for **Surviving State of Being** to understand why. If you are recovering from cancer, for example, avoiding alcohol and sugar completely has been shown to have a positive effect on the healing process. The Cancer Council now offers no safe amounts for alcohol. The harm will be most apparent in the genetically vulnerable and depleted members of our community.

SURVIVING STATE OF BEING

You may live by the 80:20 rule for food and exercise, yet you find that you never have time for yourself. For example, you eat well and exercise daily, but rarely have time to enjoy a novel, a movie, or just time to sit in your garden doing nothing at all.

Sound familiar? It may be that your boundaries aren't balanced or fully formed. Tighten these by changing the focus of your boundaries slightly. Alongside your exercise, articulate how much recovery time you will give yourself, and how this will be spent.

THRIVING STATE OF BEING

If you identify with the Thriving State of Being, it is highly likely you are good at keeping your boundaries firm and that you live by the 80:20 rule by prioritising balance in all areas of your life. However, it is easy to bleed or bend these boundaries when the pressure is on. Remember to always give back to your body by spending time restoring your energy levels. Enjoy lots of time in nature and continue to think helpful thoughts.

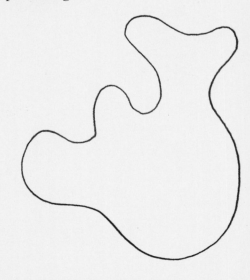

Holidays and business trips: when boundaries blur

When going on a holiday or business trip it is highly likely that you will bleed the percentage of your boundaries. You can offset any long-term effects by preparing your body beforehand for these changes. These preparation will help you recover faster, so that you won't return from your holiday needing one! (We've all been there!)

For example, if you are going on a three-week trip around Europe, it is likely you will drink and eat more than usual. For the three weeks before you leave, you may like to avoid alcohol completely and keep your diet as clean as possible. This has several advantages. Following a clean diet before leaving will give you the energy and clear-headedness that you may need as you make your way through the long list of things to complete before going away. And, if your diet has been so clean and healthy, you may not over-indulge as much, as you feel so well. It's no surprise that we tend to over-drink and eat when we're stressed. By giving yourself the space to be well, eat well, and rest well before a period of indulgence, you will most likely find that you don't need to rely on the usual 'crutch' of alcohol and fast-food to relax.

It's also important to accept that you can only do your best with what you have on hand, so don't give yourself a hard time if you do blur your boundaries temporarily.

Everything that exists in your life does so because of two things: something you did, or something you didn't do.

ALBERT EINSTEIN

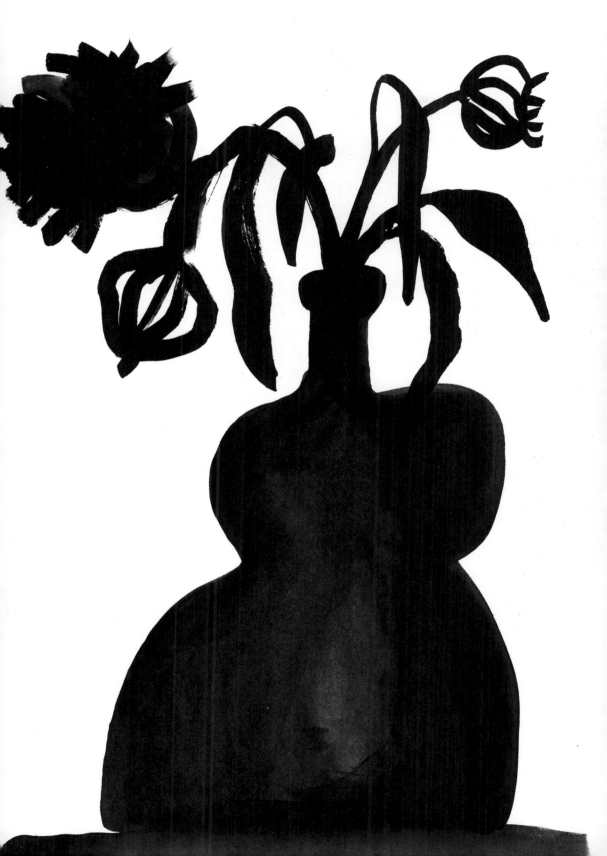

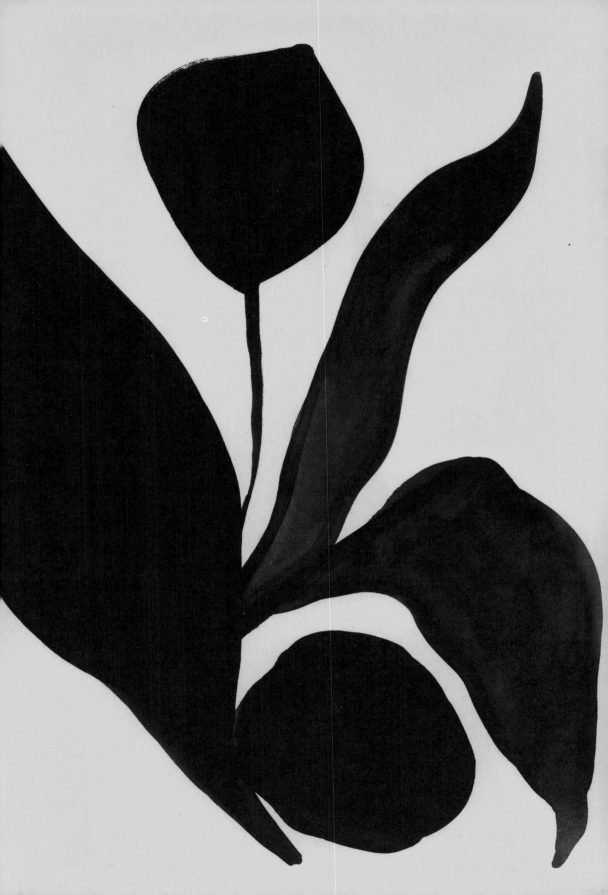

7.
STRESS AND YOUR NERVOUS SYSTEM

It's not the load
that breaks you
down, it's the way
you carry it.

LOU HOLTZ

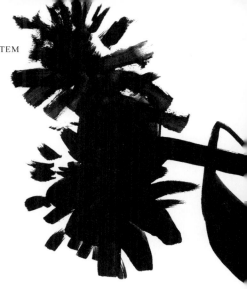

Of all the chapters in this book, this is the one that will have the most significant impact on your health and wellbeing. We invite you to read and re-read this chapter; bookmark it; highlight it; turn the pages down! We've written this chapter as a handy reference guide for your everyday life, to guide and help you on your journey.

The aim of this chapter is to help you understand and embody 'a way of being' to reduce the amount of stress hormones you may be producing. Starting right now! The impact of reducing stress hormones on your health, mental and emotional wellbeing is profound and cannot be overstated. Being able to understand, moderate and manage your nervous system is key to all positive health outcomes and has great potential to change your perspective and your life.

Let's find some space and time for you. Where you won't be interrupted. Turn off your devices. Make a cup of herbal tea, get comfortable. Now, let's take a breath and dive into one of the most important chapters in this book.

WHAT IS STRESS?

The word 'stress' refers to the physical response of the body i.e. a 'stress response'. This could easily be defined as a 'survival response'. The number-one priority for our species is survival and our body works night and day to protect us. Turning on the stress response is very easy: when given a trigger (physical danger, mental and emotional worry or distress) your body will quickly, in milliseconds, choose the survival path.

However, the body does not just turn on the stress response without stimulus. It doesn't suddenly decide 'let's get stressed!'. There needs to be a reason, such as a threat to our survival - either physically or psychologically - in order for our body to become stressed. Whenever we are exposed to a threat or danger, perceive danger, or get a shock or fright, the brain sends messages to the body to turn on the survival response. Consequently, stress hormones - like cortisol and adrenaline - enter our bloodstream.

Early humans were designed to deal with acute, life-threatening situations. Things such as finding shelter, dealing with famine and drought, war, invasion, natural disasters and the threat of an animal attack, all kept early man in a state of 'fight or flight'. Today, in comparison, we have little real danger in our day-to-day life. Most of us are fortunate enough that we are not exposed to life-threatening situations on a daily, weekly or monthly basis.

Today, for most of us, the type of stress we face regularly is long-term, ongoing **psychological or psychosocial pressure**. These pressures mean that we can literally *think ourselves into a physical stress response*. This kind of stress is associated with relationships, finances, success, parenting, children, family and global events such as the Covid-19 pandemic. Anything that leads to you to a place of worry, anger, frustration or overwhelm fits the psychological/psychosocial stress category.

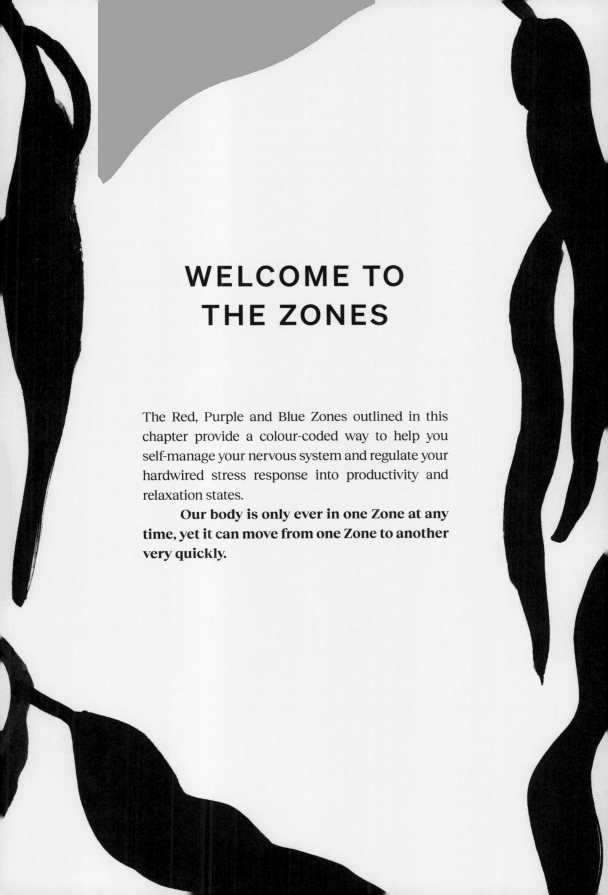

WELCOME TO THE ZONES

The Red, Purple and Blue Zones outlined in this chapter provide a colour-coded way to help you self-manage your nervous system and regulate your hardwired stress response into productivity and relaxation states.

Our body is only ever in one Zone at any time, yet it can move from one Zone to another very quickly.

Sharon's idea for colour coding the nervous system came from her friend and horsemanship mentor Angie Wicks. To provide a safe way for grooms to deal with horses coming into their training facility, Angie used the colour coding Red (for horses that are extroverted, nervous and highly reactive under pressure) and Blue (for horses that are more introverted, good thinkers and more likely to remain calm under pressure). This inspired Sharon to think about how this could be applied to humans: whether they are sympathetic reactive Red Zone or parasympathetic relaxed Blue Zone. Later came the Purple Zone, the ideal level to be in flow. Much later she became aware that others around the world also colour coded the nervous system. (Dan Bron calls this 'multiple discovery', whereby discoveries are made independently and simultaneously.) We encourage you to explore other versions of colour-coded nervous system themes. See the Resources chapter for further reading.

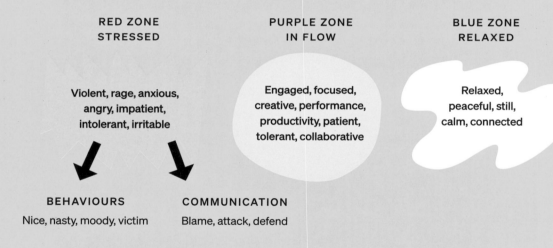

RED ZONE
STRESSED

PURPLE ZONE
IN FLOW

BLUE ZONE
RELAXED

Violent, rage, anxious,
angry, impatient,
intolerant, irritable

Engaged, focused,
creative, performance,
productivity, patient,
tolerant, collaborative

Relaxed,
peaceful, still,
calm, connected

BEHAVIOURS
Nice, nasty, moody, victim

COMMUNICATION
Blame, attack, defend

Dr Peter Parry M.B.B.S; F.R.A.N.Z.C.P, is a child and adolescent psychiatrist and a dear friend to us both. Dr Peter coined the phrase 'S for Stress' (Sympathetic) and 'P for Peace' (Parasympathetic) and has graciously given permission for the concept to be included here. Immense thanks to Dr Peter, whose work is essential to the understanding of mental health in children and adolescents, and for the compassion he shows for the human adult condition.

The Red Zone

The Sympathetic system (think 'S' for Stress), or the 'Red Zone', signals our body to be on alert when danger is real, or there is a perceived threat. This part of the nervous system activates the adrenal glands to release stress hormones into our bloodstream, which is how we may eventually arrive at adrenal fatigue (more on this later).

When you are deeply in the Red Zone, you may feel:

IMPATIENT

INTOLERANT

IRRITABLE

ANXIOUS

OVERWHELMED

ANGRY

FRUSTRATED

FEARFUL

OUT OF CONTROL

The Blue Zone

Our Parasympathetic nervous system (think 'P' for Peace), or the Blue Zone, is the rest-and-digest part of the nervous system.

When you're in the Blue Zone, you'll most likely feel:

PEACEFUL

RELAXED

CALM

REASSURED

PATIENT

LOVING

CREATIVE

CONTENT

ABLE TO GAIN PERSPECTIVE

The roles of each of these two parts of our nervous system - the Red and Blue Zones - are very different and our body cannot be in both Zones at the same time.

The Purple Zone
or 'Flow' Zone

The best, most productive way to get things done, is when you are in the Purple Zone. Although the Purple Zone is technically in the sympathetic nervous system, you have the capacity to self-regulate and maintain an ideal, steady, slow release of stress hormones. This gives you the motivation you need and yet able to enjoy a calm level of excitement to perform your tasks. We call this the Purple Zone. This is the zone for productivity and performance, its where you find 'your flow', a calm, centred approach to work, family challenges and tasks.

When you are in the Purple Zone
you may feel:

MOTIVATED

CREATIVE

FOCUSED

CALM

PATIENT

TOLERANT

CO-OPERATIVE

COLLABORATIVE

RESPECTFUL

Unpacking
the Red Zone

Imagine you wake in the morning and before you open your eyes you are already thinking about how much you have to do today. The constant background buzz of worry and mind chatter, may sound something like 'so much to do, so little time'. This kind of thinking is interpreted by the brain as threat and in milliseconds you find yourself in the Red Zone.

Really? Yes we know! Just *thinking* takes you to the Red Zone. The brain interprets messages and images from the mind continually and needs to make distinctions between safe and unsafe thoughts and images. Often your brain activates the Red Zone as though you are facing a real threat.

The brain does not know the difference between what is real and what is imagined.

Have you ever woken from a nightmare? How does it feel when you wake up? You may notice your heart rate is up, you might be shallow breathing, feeling disorientated and scared? And, yet where are you when you wake up? In bed. And, unless there is someone in the room with you that should not be there, are you safe? Yes. So it is not your physical location or reality that took you to the Red Zone, it was the mental stimulus from your subconscious or dream state. This happens in conscious states all the time; you are physically safe, yet your mind is thinking unhelpful thoughts. (More on this in Chapter 8.)

THE LIMBIC SYSTEM/MONKEY BRAIN

Depending on your thoughts and perception of situations, your brain will tell your body just how many stress hormones it needs, and how regularly these hormones will need to enter your bloodstream in order to deal with any perceived threat. The Red Zone is activated by the deeper, more primitive part of your brain, which is called the limbic system. This is often referred to by neuroscientists as the 'monkey brain'.

The limbic system/monkey brain is responsible for your continued existence, so it activates the survival (stress) response, quickly moving you into the Red Zone. In this part of a person's brain lie the following emotions: self-centredness, pessimism, anxiety, wariness and uncertainty.

When you're in the Red Zone, your thoughts may be negative and self-biased, such as 'This always happens to me'.

Once you enter the Red Zone, your adrenal glands have already begun to release the stress hormones adrenaline and cortisol into your bloodstream. The amount of stress hormones released depends on the situation and the pressure you're facing. Unrelenting pressure on the adrenal glands to produce these stress hormones may lead to a naturopathic diagnosis of adrenal exhaustion. Naturopaths and integrative medical doctors see this play out in their practice every week.

Are you in the Red Zone?

When you spend too much time in the Red Zone, your body goes through some physical changes. These include:

INCREASED HEART RATE OR HEART PALPITATIONS

HIGHER BLOOD PRESSURE

MUSCLE TENSION

FREQUENT ILLNESS

STOMACH ACHES
SLEEP DISTURBANCES
DIARRHOEA
CONSTIPATION
FATIGUE OR EXHAUSTION
HEADACHES
ACHES AND PAINS
APPETITE OR WEIGHT CHANGES

Mental and emotional signs of extended time in the Red Zone:

IRRITABILITY
IMPATIENCE
INTOLERANCE
FRUSTRATED
ANXIETY, FEAR OR WORRY
FEELING OVERWHELMED
ANGER
RAGE
VIOLENCE

Other signs include:

SADNESS
CRYING
LOSS OF PLEASURE IN EVENTS OR THINGS YOU ONCE ENJOYED
FEELINGS OF DEPRESSION
FEELING HOPELESS OR A FEELING OF HOPELESSNESS
DIFFICULTY RETAINING INFORMATION
UNWANTED REPETITIVE THOUGHTS (PARTICULARLY NEGATIVE ONES)
POOR CONCENTRATION
SCATTERED THOUGHTS AT TIMES

CASE STUDY | DR KAREN

Mary

Mary was having the week from hell. Arguments with teenage kids over curfew breaches, overdue credit card payments, and an unexpected trip out of town to deal with an elderly sick parent – and that was just last week! Ruminating on these challenging events in the supermarket, Mary was concerned to feel her breathing a little laboured.

She stopped in the fruit section and thought she felt a pain in the central part of her chest. 'Oh, no,' she thought to herself. 'I'm only 44. I can't be having a heart attack, can I?' But the pain was getting worse and a hot sweat broke out over her forehead. Fear gripped her as she left the half full trolley of groceries and headed back to her car.

Sitting in the driver's seat, the only thing she could think of was 'I've just got to get myself home. I feel like I'm going to die.' That short five-minute trip seemed to last forever. She literally fell into the foyer of her house. She managed to pick up the phone to dial for an ambulance, convinced she was in the throes of a heart attack. The pain was getting worse, there was numbness and tingling in both arms and around her lips, and Mary was having difficulty getting enough air in as the ambulance officer arrived to transport her to hospital.

Her pale and anxious appearance was convincing enough to land her in the Coronary Care Unit for 48 hours. She was poked, probed, X-rayed and then discharged. And was somewhat disappointed to see the Discharge Summary diagnosis of Acute Panic Attack, rather than Acute Myocardial Infarct.

She left the hospital with a prescription for some medication and instructions to 'take one tablet every six hours for anxiety.' For many weeks she reflected on the experience, and asked herself over and over again: 'If it was all in my head, how could I feel so bad?'

Understanding the consequences of unleashing the Red Zone is the start of regaining control of those stress hormones. In Mary's case the first domino to fall was the high stress of the urgent trip to sort out her parents.

The sleepless night of worry brought on by a wayward teenager pushed her further into the Red Zone. Fretting over the late credit card payment, and wondering about how to pay for the groceries tipped her into full-on Red Zone.

Each stressful moment, every thought Mary had, produced a surge of adrenaline and cortisol designed for survival in primitive times, but created a nightmare of symptoms in today's world. Disruption of the sympathetic (Red Zone) control room by false triggers (thoughts and perceptions) can set off the cascade of falling dominos that landed Mary in Coronary Care.

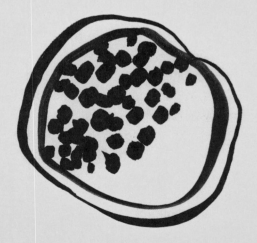

Reacting from a brain that is hijacked by a perceived danger will move you into the Red Zone. This will negatively affect behaviour, so it may not provide you with your best negotiating or communication tools. This is when you may find yourself feeling like Mary: panicky, uncertain or reactive to big and/or small issues.

Do you overact when the kids leave the fridge door ajar? Have you lost control, felt frustrated or shouted at them? This is a perfect example of a small irritation that has been made bigger because you're in the Red Zone.

When a larger quantity of these stress hormones enter your bloodstream, you may also experience irritability with feelings of frustration. An increased level of these stress hormones will often lead to anger, and eventually even rage and violence. High levels of stress hormones in your system can often mean you lose control of yourself and do or say things you may feel embarrassed about or even ashamed of later. When you move out of the Red Zone and review what happened with the value of hindsight, you may regret your behaviour.

If you're having trouble understanding what the activation of the Red Zone looks like, think about how you feel when you are in a hurry to get to a meeting or pick up the kids from school. You jump into the car and meet traffic and another person cuts in front of you. You shout or feel intense rage. This is classic Red Zone. The sense of irritation at that person and the judgement and criticism that arise in your thought process literally makes that person your enemy. At times, you may even lash out in anger.

CASE STUDY | DR KAREN

WHEN THE RED ZONE HIJACKS YOUR EMOTIONS

Sonja is a successful high-level manager, who enjoys her work and family time. She lives alone by choice but comes from a close-knit European immigrant family who live nearby. She consulted Dr Karen Coates after the following situation arose.

Sonja responded to a local radio call to attend for breast screening. Although she had only just turned 40, she presented to the mobile unit for her first ever mammogram. One of the downsides of this screening test is the potential for a false positive result. This happens when the mammogram reports a suspicious lump that eventually is found to be non-malignant. This is what happened to Sonja.

Sonja received a call-back from Breast Screen the day after her examination, asking her to see a specialist for further imaging and to go for a breast biopsy later that day. This was the start of a nightmare time, brought on, **not by the eventual results of the final tests**, but by **the hijacking of her limbic system.**

The next 24 hours were spent in extreme stress for Sonja. Broken sleep, tears and a decision not to call family or friends until she had more news, meant that Sonja dealt with her mind-demons on her own. She later recalled that she spent the night prior to the tests imagining herself in surgery, and planning how she would juggle chemotherapy around her work schedule.

In the following days, Sonja was given the welcome news that her test results were fine and there was no evidence of cancer. Instead of finding instant relief from that phone call, Sonja was stuck in the Red Zone, unable to quieten the thoughts and feelings that stemmed from that traumatic 48 hours.

She consulted me four weeks later, still in tears as she recounted her story. Her mother had been a good support during this time, but Sonja was beating herself up, trying to rationalise how she was feeling. She knew her emotional symptoms were out of proportion to reality, but she couldn't gain control of her nervous system. I spent some time explaining to her the role of the sympathetic and parasympathetic response and the role of our thoughts as a trigger for ongoing stress hormone production.

I referred her for counselling sessions with a psychologist and she sourced a local Tai Chi class as a moving meditation strategy. Once she began to realise her thoughts were the trigger, she was able to feel her way back to spending more time in the Blue Zone. As time passed, Sonja became more aware of observing her own thoughts and noticed this was the key to her becoming less reactive.

By initiating mindful practice, Sonja was able to replace her unhelpful thoughts with more helpful ones. By observing her thoughts and emotions, she was able to moderate the ancient limbic system in her brain that had previously been activating the Red Zone and driving the adrenaline pathways purely from unhelpful and catastrophising thoughts. She is continuing to enjoy her weekly Tai Chi classes.

WHAT HAPPENS TO YOUR BODY IN THE BLUE ZONE

When you're in the Blue Zone, you will retain a baseline level of the stress hormone cortisol (related to the natural circadian rhythm); however, it is physically impossible to make adrenaline in this part of our nervous system. This is a good thing!

This part of your nervous system has a very important and essential job. When you spend time in your Blue Zone your body has the best capacity to:

BUILD AND ENHANCE YOUR IMMUNE SYSTEM

PROTECT GUT MICROBIOME

IMPROVE DEEP SLEEP

IMPROVE NUTRIENT ABSORPTION

HEAL AND REPAIR ALL CELLULAR FUNCTION

ALLOW YOU TO FEEL CONTENT AND RELAXED

It's our natural state to be in the Blue Zone often.

Think of your Blue Zone time this way: your mobile phones and devices need regular recharging to work and function. **The Blue Zone, at its very essence, is your recharging and repair station.** If your phone has limited battery life it won't work. Your body is the same. If you forget to charge your phone overnight, the following day can be extremely stressful. You'll most likely spend time and energy looking for a place to recharge your phone so that it can function as you need it to.

Your body is much the same. When you're depleted or run out of energy, you will reach for caffeine, sugar, and other stimulants to push you through your fatigue. If you do not recharge your body properly, you have no residual charge to repair, heal or replenish your energy levels. You are in fact, on the road to a Depleted State of Being.

DO YOU SPEND ENOUGH TIME IN THE BLUE ZONE?

Whilst good-quality sleep is spending time in the Blue Zone, this is simply not enough. You need more time spent in rest and recovery from your busy life. This can be small pockets of time taken intermittently during your day. Long-term, you will need large chunks of time to properly restore your energy levels sufficiently. To use the phone analogy again: when your phone battery has almost run out but you only have time to recharge it for 30 minutes – you'll only get a little more use out of it before it goes completely flat. It is the same with your body. You need to take the right amount of time to recharge your battery back up to 100 per cent.

FACT!

The more you use your mobile phone, the more often you will need to recharge it. The same applies to your body. The busier you are, the more you need to go to the Blue Zone to recharge and balance your nervous system.

In today's modern world, you are continually hijacked from the Blue Zone and thrust into the Red Zone. Busy lives and pressurised situations feed unhelpful thoughts. When you catastrophise about how your day will unfold or how a person may react, you can move to the Red Zone in a millisecond. And sometimes like the story of Sonja, you can find it difficult to find your way back to the Blue Zone again.

THE PURPLE ZONE (OR FLOW ZONE)

This is the zone for productivity and performance. It's where you find your 'flow', where you're calm with a centred approach to work, family challenges and tasks. In this zone you are motivated, yet feel no irritation, impatience or intolerance. You are open to other people's ideas. You are creative and most importantly, collaborative.

Yes, you can make stress hormones, but your goal is to self-regulate, and to aim at not too much (Red Zone), not too little (Blue Zone) and end up just right (Purple Zone). Maintaining your Purple Zone when you're getting things done is the key to good health, productivity and performance throughout your daily life.

RESTING BRAIN STATE

Human beings have brain waves and a resting brain state. Similar to a resting heart rate, the resting brain state can be higher than ideal for your overall wellbeing. There are five brainwaves that change according to what you are doing and feeling. The brain state refers to the levels of brain waves and how they interact with each other.

An elevated resting brain state signals a nervous system that is constantly on guard. In this agitated state, the nervous system is ready to jump to the Red Zone at the slightest provocation.

Are you 'wired, but tired'?
You can't switch off and find it hard to rest and relax?

Do you find it hard to rest and relax without feeling the need to do something else, whether it's physical or mental? When a person has an elevated resting brain state, it is more challenging to enter the Blue Zone to relax. You will also have a reduced ability to maintain the Purple Zone where you can be productive. Spending more time in the Blue Zone is the prescription for reducing your resting brain state.

DO YOU SPEND ENOUGH TIME IN THE PURPLE ZONE?

Remember Goldilocks and the Three Bears? She doesn't want too much; she doesn't want too little; she just wants the right amount. Like most of us, Goldilocks was searching for the Purple Zone.

When you're in the Purple Zone it can be a good idea to set a timer for 40 minutes. After 40 minutes, take a break, have a stretch, drink some water and dip into the Blue Zone. Then you can return to your task. Taking this break will ensure you don't slide into the other direction towards the unproductive Red Zone.

YOU'VE GOT A FRIEND IN ME

The good news is the Blue and Purple Zone have a very good friend: this is the most modern part of your brain, called the prefrontal lobe. This part of your brain, what we call the 'CEO', can help you moderate and manage your monkey brain. This helps to keep you out of your Red Zone and allows you to maintain your status within the Purple Zone. It is through the activation of the CEO/prefrontal lobe that we witness some of our best human traits.

The CEO, along with the social part of your brain, allows you to be optimistic, collaborative, creative, curious and open to others. The CEO allows you to handle complex tasks, including higher-order learning and, most importantly, be philosophical about life and the lessons you learn through facing adversity.

The activation of your CEO and social brain helps you to switch back into the Blue Zone. When this occurs, your body will feel safe, and you'll become more emotionally intelligent and aware. This allows you to connect deeply with others and experience a heightened awareness of purpose and meaning, where you'll feel love and affection for life, and be open to falling in love.

Neurological imaging of Buddhist monks who meditate regularly show increased activation and size of the prefrontal lobe. This CEO part of our brain acts as the moderator to the entire human system including the Blue Zone, and seems to be the pathway to more peaceful feelings.

TAKE NOTE

The amount of alcohol you drink in one sitting has a profound effect on the ability of your prefrontal cortex to act as the 'CEO' and be the regulator of the monkey brain. Increased chronic, long-term consumption of alcohol causes a shrinkage of the prefrontal cortex. This can explain why we may feel shaky or sometimes paranoid and insecure after a heavy boozing session. More worryingly, more serious long-term health issues can occur.

In the Red Zone, we make more mistakes yet we seem not to notice until others bring this to our attention; if we are still in the Red Zone we may not respond kindly to them – we may also act overly controlling and authoritative.

Learning to activate the CEO part of your brain more often will allow you to moderate and manage the limbic monkey brain. The more you use the CEO, the stronger the neurological connections in this part of your brain become, producing super highways, allowing you to access these regulatory pathways faster.

Ring any bells?

- Do you believe that stress is a constant, irritable force in your life?

- Do you constantly think: 'If everyone does everything I want them to do perfectly, in my time, to my specifications, I will not be stressed.'

- Do you believe that you're stressed due to deadlines or tasks that others expect you to do, or ask you to perform?

The reality? People and the demands of life are going to upset you, put pressure on you and generally piss you off! Sadly, there is no magical pill or one thing that can make life's challenges and tasks disappear.

Integrating and assessing how stress affects different parts of you is your first step to returning your body and mind to the Purple and Blue Zones.

The only thing you can control is how you react or respond to a challenge.

You can't prevent or change the weather, yet you can dress appropriately for it.

Sometimes it's the most capable and successful women who push the boundaries of stress and stressors, who have a much harder time finding their Blue Zone. Living with constant pressure and stress has become so normal to them, they may not even notice it anymore. If their tribe and everyone around them is in the same hurried state, this also supports the theory that this way of living and feeling is normal. If this sounds familiar, you are most likely living in the **Survival State of Being**. You may feel healthy and proactive, until the wheels fall off.

CASE STUDY | DR KAREN

Emily

I remember a discussion with one of Australia's most successful designers in the fashion industry. Here was a woman who existed on six hours sleep a night, rarely took more than a long weekend for a vacation and was available for her business seven days per week. She felt well and energised by her passion for her business, but wanted to know whether her body was coping with what was a huge work demand.

My first thought was that this woman had an incredibly positive attitude to life and was surrounded by like-minded colleagues. She had no financial stress in her life and contributed to her community both financially and through mentoring women starting out in her industry. But her work/life balance was not right. My fears were confirmed when she went on to mention that her periods had been absent for several months. As she was in her early 40s, she was too early for a normal menopause. In women, this can be a strong signal that the physical body is not keeping up with an incredibly busy body and productive mind.

WHAT HAPPENS TO YOUR BODY WHEN YOU'RE STRESSED

As you've now read, when your brain registers a threat, either internally (triggered by thinking or perceiving) or externally (from a person or situation), it prepares your body to fight, flight, freeze or faint (the Red Zone). During this response, your body prioritises its own physiological functions to direct all its energy towards establishing safety and therefore meet the ultimate human species priority, survival.

Adrenaline is the short-term response; it creates urgency and gives your body the ability to run or fight. When it is released into the bloodstream, your heart rate and blood pressure increase, blood sugar is released from the liver to provide energy, breathing becomes rapid and shallow in order to get oxygen to the muscles quickly, your mental focus becomes alert but narrow (black/white), and blood flow is prioritised to your arms and legs to give you the ability to move quickly and protect yourself.

These changes enable you to respond quickly to danger. However, when adrenaline is produced and you are not in physical danger the physical affects can produce a panic attack (as demonstrated by Mary's story earlier) and lead to long-term anxiety as well as increase your baseline cortisol levels.

THE ROLE OF CORTISOL

Cortisol, on the other hand, is designed to keep you alive during long-term stress. Historically, times of war or invasion, famine and drought raised the levels of this stress hormone. Cortisol instructs the body to slow down the metabolism and to eat (particularly sugar and carbs) so that it can store fat in preparation for the perceived famine or harsh environment.

Overeating due to elevated cortisol levels encourages the body to store fat around the waist, back and tummy. It also interferes with fat burning and the ability to control body composition, often leading to complications such as metabolic syndrome. Tackling excess cortisol levels is paramount to successful body fat loss. See the solutions in the next chapter, Stress Resilience, where we outline the keys to reducing cortisol levels.

Elevated cortisol sets you on a mental path of worry. Historically, this would help you find solutions to food shortages. Today, this constant mental activity leads to overthinking and anxiety, increasing our internal pressure and making you less stress resilient. To cope with external pressure, we may self-medicate with food, alcohol, drugs, overwork, over exercise or seek pharmaceutical support.

Sometimes this unresolved internal pressure and overstressed body can affect you so deeply - mentally and emotionally - that self-loathing and a regular destructive internal dialogue becomes the norm. This adds to the psychological stress, and so the cycle continues.

Stress hormones dramatically increase chronic inflammation in the body. Chronic inflammation is the mechanism that drives most of the lifestyle diseases, as inflammation also changes the epigenetic landscape of cells and shortens telomeres. Find more on this in Chapter 12.

STRESS AND YOUR IMMUNE SYSTEM

Unmanaged pressure that leads to a stressed body has an effect on your immune system. When your limbic/monkey brain tells your adrenal glands to prioritise the production of stress hormones, this interferes with the building and supporting of your immune system and baseline reproductive hormones. This means your immune system is not at its optimal level, leaving you susceptible to external threats such as colds, flus, viruses and contributing to the risk of internal cellular dysfunctions such as cancer. Worryingly the epigenetic changes created by chronic stress can be inherited by future generations.

When elevated to chronic levels, cortisol also interrupts the production of other hormones (including the sleep hormone melatonin). A lack of melatonin can cause poor sleep quality and in turn the stress of insomnia increases cortisol levels even more. It's a nasty, vicious cycle.

Cortisol is an energy regulator. Think of it as the person who maintains rations until help arrives. Only priorities for survival will be given precious calories until the danger passes and cortisol levels reduce.

In your body, one of the lowest priorities is the production of collagen; this means that long-term stress has a catastrophic influence on your skin and hair, causing more wrinkles and sagging skin earlier in life.

In today's fast-paced technological world, the stress response is being switched on for non-life-threatening, emotive reasons. Internal and external pressure is driving your monkey brain into a survival response and your body is reacting as if you were in acute danger when you are physically safe (like an awake nightmare).

It's important to understand and recognise your reactivity and learn how to manage the monkey brain. Unless you intervene, the limbic/monkey part of your brain will hijack your body into producing stress hormones more often than necessary.

The good news is, it is possible to retrain your brain and learn to be productive and get things done - without becoming stressed. We cover this in the next chapter; we encourage you to finish reading this one first.

WHY YOU NEED TO DE-STRESS

Our bodies are not designed to spend too much time in the Red Zone. Think of the Red Zone as the emergency lane, complete with flashing lights and warning signals. Spending too much time in the Red Zone means your physical, mental and emotional balance deteriorates.

YOUR BODY IN THE RED ZONE

The stress response was audited in a study on, of all things, bungee jumpers. To measure the hormones produced in this risky activity, researchers took baseline samples of the stress hormone family – including adrenaline and cortisol – along with markers of immune function. They measured the participants levels immediately before and after a 60-metre bungee jump.

The researchers found that:

- Stress hormones surged in seconds (as expected).

- The elevated stress hormones from the bungee jump caused the immune system to falter for around 48 hours after the jump, affecting the body's ability to fight bacterial infections.

- The euphoria of the jump was directly related to the jumper's ability to produce a 'natural high' hormone called β-endorphin. (This natural high hormone could be referred to as home-made morphine. It's no wonder exercise can be addictive for some.)

- Other blood indicators confirmed that this active **SYMPATHETIC** response (i.e. the Red Zone) was catabolic. This means tissue was broken down in the body rather than replenished. This type of response cannot go on forever, or the body starts to break down.

ARE YOU THINKING YOURSELF STRESSED?

Every day your thoughts and perceptions are racing. Are you paying enough attention to what is happening in your body?

Whilst you are living your busy life, your brain and body are working very hard to keep up with your 'to do' or 'to be' list. It's likely that your body often considers itself to be in 'danger'. Your body then responds by looking after its survival. The truth is: we are rarely in actual danger; we just think that way as the amygdala (the emotional, fear sensor) within the monkey brain is perceiving danger.

OUR THOUGHTS HAVE MEANING AND CONSEQUENCES

As a result, your thoughts can hijack your body into the Red Zone. For instance, if your brain (remember the brain does not know the difference between what is real and what is imagined or perceived) considers a situation to be unsafe, that signal is then transmitted to your body. Being in this state for weeks, months or years is exhausting. While most of us are able to keep going, it tends to be due to coffee, sugar and adrenaline. Without these stimulants, you're left only with deep exhaustion.

Research has shown us that long-term elevated stress hormones are the greatest contributor to the development of most medical diseases.

Remind yourself every day that your body is not a machine. It is a biological living organism with its own innate wisdom. If you give your body what it needs, it has an enormous capacity to self-regulate.

When you can maintain your nervous system in the Purple Zone while getting things done and then actively recharge and recover in the Blue Zone, you will have found the key to sustainability in life.

IT'S ALL ABOUT YOU

Top on your list of priorities should be your own health, your own time and your own space. Commonly called 'me time', this involves more than just good, healthy food and regular exercise. It also includes managing your nervous system, so that you spend time in your Blue Zone to allow your body to rest and recover.

Think you don't have the time to relax?
Let's look at it another way. Do you have time to be ill?

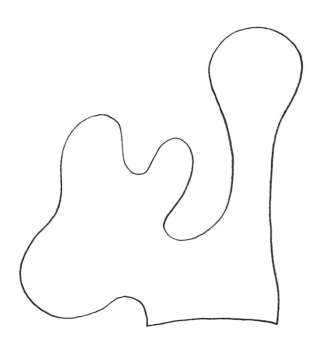

Make time to take care of yourself or make time to be sick.

DR ROSS WALKER

INTEGRATIVE CARDIOLOGIST

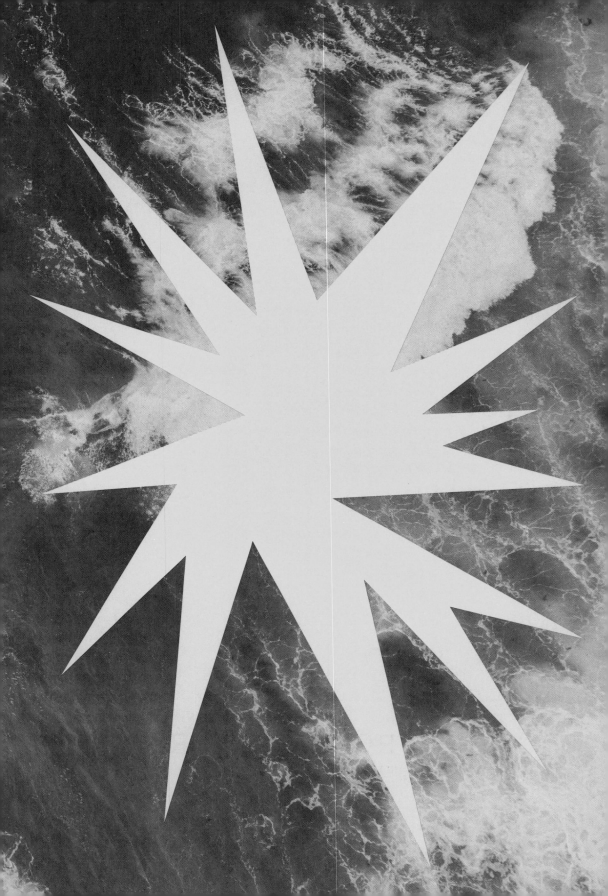

If your health fails, or your mental and emotional wellbeing is less than optimum, everything around you will most likely be compromised: your career, family, finances… the list goes on. Your health and wellbeing is the most precious of jewels and should be guarded and nurtured to ensure you are well and thriving. Self-preservation is selfless rather than selfish, because being at your optimal health level, whatever that may be, is the best gift you can offer to yourself and everyone in your life.

We have met thousands and thousands of women over the last three decades in our individual careers, many who have tried to negotiate with their body to push boundaries beyond its capabilities. Sadly, many of them have ended up with a medical label of disease or are mentally and emotionally exhausted.

What we have witnessed in the vast majority of women is a trend of living mainly in the Purple and Red Zones. Many people both men and women, do not spend enough time in Blue Zone. Your body needs to recover and repair, otherwise something will break down.

Pay attention to the warning signs in your own body.

Would you ignore a red flashing light on the dash of your car? Imagine if you put a business card over the flashing light because it is irritating you. Before long, the car will come to a grinding halt. The car repairs may be a lot more expensive than if you had stopped and paid attention when the light first began flashing. Your body is the same, it needs you to listen and do a little before you need to do a lot.

Are you being honest with yourself?

When asked, 'How do you *really* feel?', many women will often be reduced to tears. If they honestly allow themselves to feel, sobs will wrack their body. So many women are quite terrified to look at the reality of what emotions and feelings lie under the surface. There seems to be an irrational fear of failure, a belief that 'I should be able to do this'. This fear is compounded by the fact that many of their friends and family are in this state. Therefore, it must be normal!

The most worrying part about this abnormal stressed state is that we are teaching our children that this State of Being is normal. In fact, this is not normal; this is the survival response. Children learn from what they experience. As women we can shift our perspective to what is sustainable, not only for our benefit, for our children's benefit as well.

Let's be honest.

It is here, in this place of transparency, where your best work is done. Once you realise and acknowledge a real or potential problem, with this acknowledgement there can be no more denial. Change, healing and recovery can begin.

Listen to your body.

ARE YOU SLEEPING WELL?

DO YOU FEEL IRRITATED?

DO YOU LACK PATIENCE AND TOLERANCE?

ARE YOU EASILY IRRITATED AND FRUSTRATED?

IS YOUR IMMUNE SYSTEM DEPLETED?

DO YOU CRAVE SUGAR?

DO YOU EMOTIONALLY EAT?

Our body clearly has some non-negotiables. Spending time in the Blue Zone is a major one. Read on to explore how to include Blue Zoning in your life as a stress resilience tool.

Just because you can do something, doesn't mean you should take the task on.

WHEN AND WHERE TO SEEK HELP

Some situations, such as a job in emergency services, or being trapped in a domestic violence situation, can expose very real dangers. In the event of domestic violence, supportive help is essential not just from family, but also from the police or family and domestic violence services. If you work in emergency services, you should receive training to help moderate and manage natural Red Zone urges. However, these jobs are also supported by counsellors and psychologists following harrowing or life-threatening moments. We encourage you to gain access to these essential avenues of support. See the Resources section for where to seek help.

In the next chapter, we unpack how we can still tick our boxes and manage to get things done without compromising our health. In other words, how do we as women become stress resilient? Read on to learn how to manage the greatest irritant of all, the mind.

HOW TO ENTER THE BLUE ZONE

What does it feel like to be in the Blue Zone? Mostly you'll feel relaxed, calm, centred, connected, creative, joyous, content, open, loving and accepting. Being in the Blue Zone is about parasympathetic nervous system activation. It's not about physically moving and producing the endorphins you get from enjoying a run, exercise, hobby or sport. These are good activities that produce a very different outcome in the body. The Blue Zone is about **stopping, resting and digesting.**

Our body deals better with a stress response in short bouts, followed by long recovery. Think of stress in terms of short sprints, rather than a marathon. Try to find moments in your day to briefly dip into Blue Zone moment. Here are some ideas:

- Take ten deep breaths when you visit the bathroom.
- Practice deep breathing as you drive the car (on the way to work or school pickup).
- Set your alarm to remind you to take a short five-minute break from your screen every 90 minutes. Do some deep breathing.
- Burn a calming aromatherapy oil (such as chamomile, Melissa, lavender, jasmine, sweet basil, bergamot or valerian, or a blend of these).
- Play calming music while you work or drive.
- Set your screensaver to display inspirational quotes.

DIAPHRAGMATIC BREATHING:
A SIMPLE WAY TO GET INTO THE BLUE ZONE

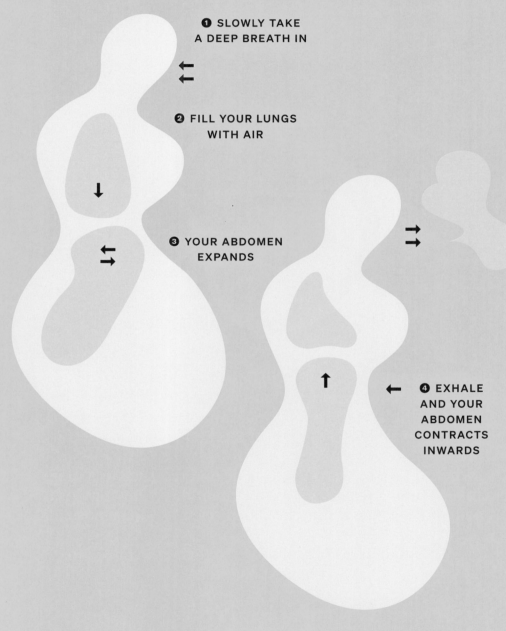

❶ SLOWLY TAKE A DEEP BREATH IN

❷ FILL YOUR LUNGS WITH AIR

❸ YOUR ABDOMEN EXPANDS

❹ EXHALE AND YOUR ABDOMEN CONTRACTS INWARDS

IF YOU'RE STUCK IN THE RED ZONE

It is highly likely you will still find yourself in the Red Zone from time to time. The trick is to know when you are in that Zone. It's also hugely important to know how to find your 'off switch'.

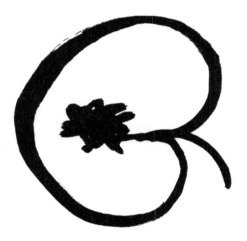

Being in the Red Zone will happen from time to time, so be kind to yourself. What's important is recognising when you are in the Red Zone, and having the tools to recover from this state.

When you have left the Red Zone and returned to a more manageable Purple Zone, implement the following tips to help move yourself into the Blue Zone as soon as possible.

We unpack further solutions to Red Zone hijack in the next chapter.

RED ZONE EXIT STRATEGIES

1.

If possible, remove yourself from the Red Zone trigger.

2.

Use positive messages to remind yourself
that this phase will pass.

3.

Learn how to moderate and manage your reactions through
diaphragmatic breathing.

4.

Practise switching from unhelpful thoughts to helpful
(see page 293 for some suggestions).

We strongly recommend you seek the support of
a trained professional if you find yourself overwhelmed
in the Red Zone.

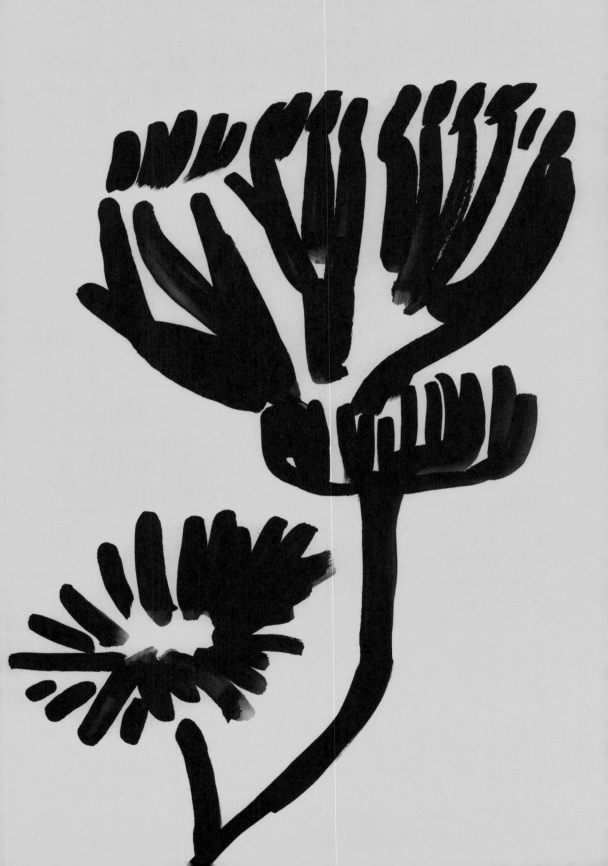

8.
BUILDING STRESS RESILIENCE

If you are depressed, you are living in the past; If you are anxious, you are living in the future; If you are at peace, you are living in the present.

LAO TZU

How do you deal with the day to day pressures of modern life? How can you manage the relationship with yourself and others so you can be in the Blue Zone more often? Let's deconstruct pressure to understand a bit more about how to manage it.

We see two types of pressure in modern life, internal and external.

INTERNAL PRESSURE

Internal pressure is related to your thoughts and feelings; how you think about yourself in relation to others and the world, and the expectations you may place on yourself in so many ways. This is often referred to as your 'internal dialogue'.

You will have more conversations with yourself throughout your life than with anybody else.

EXTERNAL PRESSURE

External pressure relates to deadlines, family responsibilities, timelines, external expectations, and finances - to name just a few! These are the pressures that exist outside of your internal world.

No matter what the pressure - internal or external - how you think about what is happening to you will have the potential to pull you into the Red Zone.

UNPACKING INTERNAL PRESSURE

While you may think no one is listening to your thoughts, your brain is. Your brain interprets your internal dialogue and files these thoughts into two categories: safety and threat. The resulting messages communicated to your body via your nervous system will activate the Blue, Purple or Red Zones (as covered in Chapter 7). This process occurs every millisecond of your life.

Time to check in.
How often do you think unhelpful
or angry thoughts?

Have you ever noticed that you do not need anyone around you to get yourself mentally or emotionally worked up? One catastrophising or angry thought and suddenly... you're in the Red Zone.

Being aware of how you are thinking is a major key to managing your nervous system. *How* you think about what is happening to you is much more important than *what is* actually happening to you.

Remember the nightmare story in Chapter 7?
It's a reminder that the brain does not know the difference
between what is real and what is imagined or perceived.

VISUALISATION AND INTERNAL PRESSURE

Read the following visualisation. Then close your eyes for a moment and concentrate, focusing your attention on the pictures in your mind. The clearer the pictures, the better the experiment.

'Imagine you are holding a lemon in your hand. In your mind, peel the lemon and notice how juicy the lemon is. Juice runs onto your hand and you can smell the strong aroma of the lemon. Now, imagine bringing the lemon up to your mouth and bite into the flesh. The juice runs down your chin, your mouth is filled with juice and it tastes very sour and bitter. As you swallow the juice, your mouth is left with the aftertaste of a very sour lemon.'

You may notice you are salivating – the brain constantly sends signals to the body, relaying information about what we are thinking, and the feelings and emotions these thoughts create. When you imagine eating a lemon, your brain sends signals to your body to provide the saliva, along with the enzymes needed to help digest it, even though you only imagined the food – you are not actually eating a lemon.

Unhelpful thoughts can have the brain sending messages to the body to be on high alert: a threat or danger is coming or is present. And here's the kicker, you could be sitting in a park on a beautiful day, with no actual physical threat in sight yet your internal world may be worrying and imagining and in response your body will be swimming in stress hormones.

Put simply, whatever the mind perceives, the body believes. This is a vital element in understanding and managing your nervous system.

The subconscious, via the brain, pushes the body into a Red Zone stress response based on the mind's visions. This is because the monkey brain takes the mind – both conscious and subconscious – at face value. It does not self-actualise and think 'This is a dream' or 'I am imagining this'.

THOUGHTS, FEELINGS AND EMOTIONS

We have already discovered how thoughts can affect your body and activate the Red Zone. When you pay more attention to what you are thinking as the 'observer' of your thoughts, you become more conscious and aware. You'll also have a greater ability to listen to your internal dialogue, auditing your thoughts as they happen.

Imagine if you were to pay full attention to your thoughts for one hour; you are granted the magical ability to pluck your thoughts from your mind one-by-one. Now imagine two buckets to put these thoughts into: one bucket is for helpful thoughts; the other for unhelpful thoughts. At the end of the hour, which one of your buckets would be more full?

In our experience, the vast majority of people say their thoughts would fill the unhelpful bucket faster. However, this is where the eternal problem of psychological and psychosocial stress lies. Your thoughts influence your brain; in response, your brain sends a message to your body to stay in the Blue Zone or to push you into the Red Zone.

WAKING UP TO STRESS
THE FOLLOWING THOUGHT PATTERN MAY SOUND FAMILIAR TO SOME.

Julie woke one morning and thought about the day ahead. While she lay in bed, her thoughts became unhelpful and worrying: 'How am I going to get through this day today? I have so much to do and so little time. I am already tired. I didn't have a great sleep. I can't wait for the day to finish. It is going to be a hard and difficult day. I hope I can get through it.'

Now imagine you are the brain and you need to decide what to tell the body. You have two choices: is the day ahead safe or unsafe? If you answered 'unsafe', you are right.

Based on this kind of 'unsafe' thinking your brain will be cautious. Your body will be told: 'You are about to meet some threats ahead, be prepared.' Your body then prepares by activating the Red Zone in case of danger, and the waking nightmare begins.

Julie jumps out of bed, and walks, naked, into the bathroom and catches sight of herself in the full-length mirror. Will Julie think helpful or unhelpful thoughts?

Julie thinks:
'Why am I too fat/skinny/saggy/too short/tall? I wish I was... '. She hops into the shower and continues with her destructive unhelpful thinking. 'How did this happen? I don't have time to take care of myself. I have too many things to do and everyone relies on me. I hold it all together, and I am exhausted. No wonder I am such a mess. How can anyone be attracted to this body?'

What have we learned from Julie? Will her brain interpret her thinking as safe or unsafe? Before Julie had even stepped out of her bedroom, her internal pressure is on the increase. Her stress hormones rise and increase in intensity. Before she had even begun her day, her thoughts were causing her internal pressure to rise, tipping her into the Red Zone.

Now it's your turn.
Ask yourself these two questions:

QUESTION ONE

If your **internal pressure** is high from unhelpful thoughts, how much **external pressure** can you manage?

ANSWER

With stress hormones already in your bloodstream from your unhelpful thinking, you will have less capacity to deal with any external pressures in your upcoming day.

QUESTION TWO

Which type of **pressure** do you have more control over: **internal** or **external**?

ANSWER

Internal pressure. When you manage your thoughts, you also manage your nervous system.

THE SELF-MANAGEMENT STRESS PYRAMID

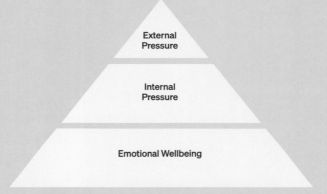

At the top of the pyramid and the smallest wedge is **External Pressure**. The least amount of control you have is external; 2020 was a great lesson in how little control each of us has of our external world.

The middle wedge **Internal Pressure** is larger. You have more control of how you think about yourself and how you mentally frame the challenges you face in life. A thought can be deconstructed into 'true' or 'false', and thoughts can also be changed. In fact, the single most powerful self-management tool you have (no matter what challenges you face) is to choose a better, solution-based thought.

The base, and biggest wedge, of the pyramid is your **Emotional Wellbeing**. This is because our emotional state is the foundation that supports us to manage any kind of stress, uncertainty and self-doubt. Have you ever noticed when you feel emotionally bruised or wounded you have less capacity to manage any kind of pressure? This is why we have included the chapter on Emotional Wellbeing in this book as well as recommending those who feel emotionally overwhelmed seek professional support from a trained emotional or mental health specialist.

You have around 25,000 to 70,000 thoughts a day.

BALANCING INTERNAL AND EXTERNAL PRESSURES

Unhelpful thoughts increase your internal pressure. Why is this? Because your brain does not know the difference between what is real or what is perceived. If your internal pressure is unmanaged, thinking unhelpful thoughts means you will have less tolerance, patience and energy to deal with external pressures. In order to understand how to manage your internal pressure, let's look more deeply into the mind to understand how thoughts can be brought to 'heal'.

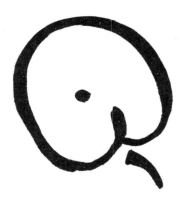

Lessons from Mr Wong

Many years ago, when she was in her 30s, Sharon found herself in a very dark place. The end of a relationship, and subsequent financial pressures as a single Mum brought on a sadness and depression that overwhelmed her. After wallowing in self-pity for many years and contemplating ending the pain forever, she decided that she needed to live for her daughter, Sarah, who was about eight years old at the time. Sharon's empathy for Sarah was her first step on her own path to find inner peace. This empathy dragged her back from the brink of despair where the monkey brain had her firmly in its grasp. In fact the monkey, she says, had become an overpowering gorilla.

One of the most healing parts of her journey to inner peace was learning the practice of Qi Gong. After learning the fundamentals, she decided to train with an older Chinese man who taught her more that she imagined possible.

'This beautiful and powerful practice had a huge influence on the way I lived. It gave me the opportunity to experience life from a different perspective. Qi Gong was one of the most important things I have ever done for myself.

'I was a busy fitness professional running on adrenaline; a single Mum barely making ends meet. I was also depressed.

'At first, Qi Gong totally challenged my patience and tolerance (i.e. I had none and it gave me some!). This newfound patience allowed me to slow down enough, until yoga, and eventually seated meditation became more appealing to me. Without these three extraordinary practices I would not be the person I am today; transformed from a depressed victim into a grateful loving woman.

'They say the teacher will arrive when the student is ready. I believe each of us need to embrace being a student of these magnificent ancient arts to find the essence of self.

'I remember meeting Mr. Wong through a friend and asking him if he could help me with my Qi Gong practice. He agreed, and we met by the side of a river for my first personal lesson. He watched patiently as I went through Shibashi, the series of 18 movements that coordinate movement with breathing and concentration. I thought I executed each move perfectly. He looked at me when I had finished and said, "Busy mind."

'I was shocked and confused. How on earth could he know that, and how dare he say it! Yet, he knew. And deep down, I also knew it was true. With a background in choreography, I had perfected the movements, yet they were performed on autopilot. What was lacking was my intention and attention. Instead of focusing, my mind was wondering what he would say, and what I had to do later that day.

'This moment gave rise to a discussion about "mind", because at that stage in my life, I thought I was my mind. Today, I know it was my mind that was causing me so much suffering.

'Mr. Wong asked me: "Can you change your mind?" My answer was: "Yes, of course." Mr Wong said: "So if you can change your mind... then who are you?"

'This profound question was the end of my first lesson. During the following week until my next lesson, this question played on my mind. My next lesson began with me asking Mr. Wong: "If I am not my mind, then who am I?". His answer was simple: "This is why you are here in physical form, to explore and self-enquire."

'Weeks later I was still grappling with the original question. We had a discussion that went something along the lines of the following conversation:

Sharon	'Mr. Wong I am struggling with my mind. I feel confused by realising I am not my mind, yet can't really understand what it means.'
Mr. Wong	'Hold up your arm. Are you this arm?'
Sharon	'Yes.'
Mr. Wong	'Is it all of you?"
Sharon	'No.'
Mr. Wong	'So, like our arm, our mind is not all of us, it is a part of us. It is associated with our ego; it is the conditioned aspect of our awareness. Find balance by observing [your] mind.'
Sharon	'How?'
Mr. Wong	'Can you move your arm, bend it, shake the hand, squeeze a fist at will?'
Sharon	'Yes.'
Mr. Wong	'Do you have as much control over your mind?'
Sharon	'No. It drives me crazy and I think terrible things about myself.'
Mr. Wong	'You can choose to stop doing that.'
Sharon	'How?'
Mr. Wong	'By practising how to manage your mind by doing Qi Gong and observing your mind with meditation.'

'Qi Gong put me on the path to slowing down my mind and noticing my senses and the sensations in my body. The first time I became physically aware of my Qi (energy or life force), I was in love with life. I realised that we are so much more than our busy minds.'

It's only a thought, and a thought can be changed.

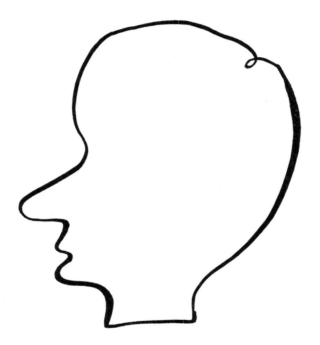

One inspirational person who has mastered a challenging and difficult situation is Nelson Mandela. He said he became the master of his thoughts by focusing on finding the good in every situation he faced during his time on Robben Island. He realised his captors controlled his physical environment and he had no control over how he was treated. Inspired by the poem Invictus by William Earnest Henley, he realised his captors did not have control over his mind. He could choose his own thoughts at will.

THE FOUR LEVELS OF THOUGHT

A simple way to break down your thoughts is to cognitively practise how to consciously audit them. The very practice of interrupting your thought process is a wonderful way to create new synapses in the brain to rewire this activity.

PURE THOUGHTS
PRODUCTIVE THOUGHTS

(ABOVE THE LINE HELPFUL THOUGHTS)

(BELOW THE LINE UNHELPFUL THOUGHTS)

NON-PRODUCTIVE THOUGHTS
DESTRUCTIVE THOUGHTS

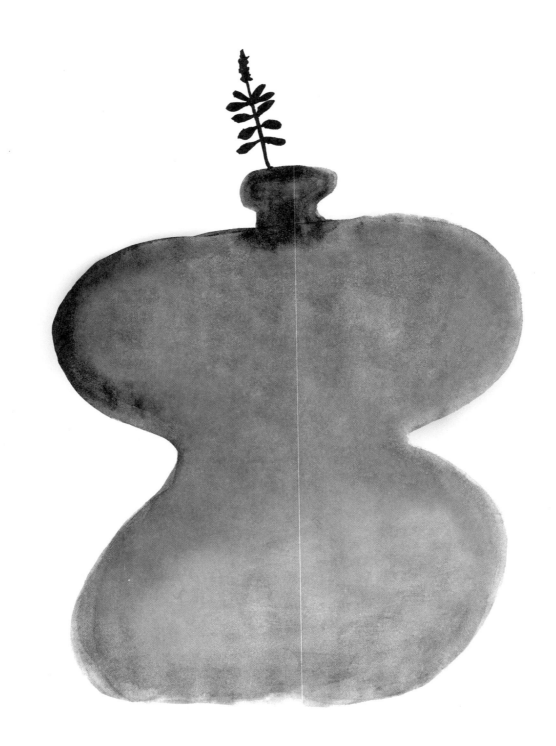

UNHELPFUL THOUGHTS

DESTRUCTIVE THOUGHTS

Let's start with the lowest level of thought. These are thoughts such as: 'What a stupid thing to do/say. I am too old. I will never be as fit as that. My legs are too short. My life is horrible, everyone is so much luckier than me. I am not lovable/successful. If only I could do that.' (You get the idea!)

Destructive thoughts do little to make you successful or feel good about yourself. They can undermine your self-esteem and exacerbate feelings of uncertainty and doubt. Whenever you find yourself thinking destructive thoughts, this is the time to use your awareness to audit those thoughts by shifting them into a more supportive internal dialogue.

NON-PRODUCTIVE THOUGHTS

These thoughts are usually related to circle thinking. We've all been there. When you overthink a certain situation – your internal message(s) make you feel that there is not another solution or answer other than to worry.

Often, non-productive thoughts can be related to something that has happened in your past, that is unable to be changed. Remember: *Nothing that has happened in the past can ever be changed, no matter how hard you try.* Focusing on past experiences only directs your attention into a void of nothingness; it brings hurt and pain into sharp focus; it highlights any loss or anger.

Some people do suffer from post-traumatic stress disorder (PTSD). If this is you, we highly recommend you seek professional counselling. And don't lose hope. Even those who have suffered from PTSD can experience post-traumatic growth (PTG). Professional counselling and being aware of your thought processes can help you find some solutions and lessons from your past situation. With every trauma – no matter how big, there will be some element of good – no matter how small.

HELPFUL THOUGHTS

PRODUCTIVE THOUGHTS

Productive thought is solution-based thinking. We recommend that you use this kind of thinking to create and navigate obstacles in life.

Rather than focusing on why or what can't be done (which leads you back to negative thought patterns), productive thought is intuitive and opens many possibilities. It involves 'thinking outside the square' and judging possible outcomes in a positive way. It's about invention, production and finding solution. This way of thinking supports your self-esteem and encourages you to have hope and feel happier overall.

American author and humourist Erma Bombeck wrote: 'Worry is like a rocking chair – it gives you something to do but it never gets you anywhere.' Instead of ruminating on your fears or struggles, turn your mind to the question: 'Is there anything I can do about this right now?'

This is typical productive thinking: focus on the things you can change and control, and let go of, or accept what is out of your control.

PURE THOUGHTS

This way of thinking includes thoughts of love, peace, happiness, gratitude, thankfulness, compassion and forgiveness, to name just a few. Pure thoughts allows you to be completely at peace with yourself and the world. It encourages you to see the connection to yourself, and to build a caring relationship with others, based on self-acceptance and love.

By being in this place of pure thought you will be able to understand that not everyone you know is as emotionally free as you now are. This is important – from this place you will be in a position to offer compassion and empathy for their emotional pain. This can pave the way to forgiveness. Pure thought is the level that raises humanity's consciousness – a collective hope for everyone to benefit.

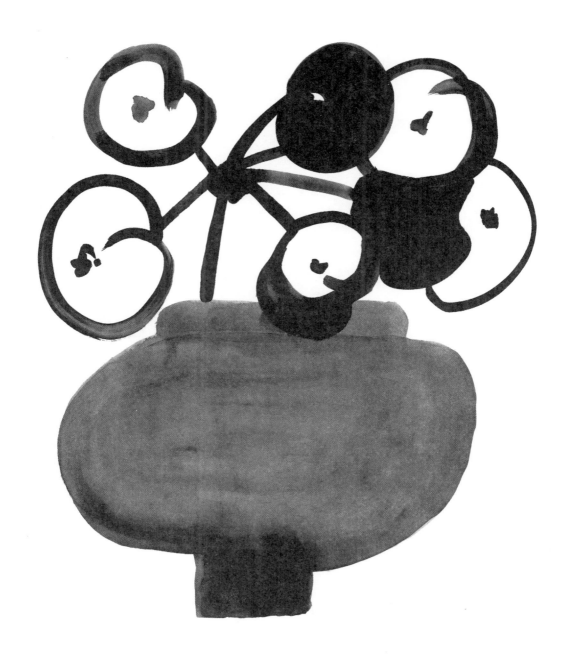

The perfect world
is created when
the mind is free
to see it.

BYRON KATIE

THE FOUR LEVELS OF THOUGHT AND YOUR NERVOUS SYSTEM

These four levels of thought can be categorised into the following buckets: helpful and unhelpful (see Chapter 7 for a reminder about your buckets).

Your helpful buckets contain productive and pure thoughts; your unhelpful buckets hold any destructive and non-productive thoughts (and it's these thoughts that will push you into the Red Zone). We need more productive thoughts in our thought bucket every day. Although it is not an exact science, it is the productive thoughts that assist you to stay in the Purple Zone.

So how can you weed out your unhelpful thoughts? It can sound daunting but there's a simple script we like to follow.

Rather than:
'I can't do this, it's too hard.' (A non-productive thought.)

Think:
'That is an unhelpful thought (insert your own name). Do you have a helpful thought?' (A productive thought process.)

Try it! Rather than going down the negative path, you will instead shift to the smoother path of 'flow'. Rather than wasting your time and energy on irritation, impatience, anger and frustration, you literally tell your non-productive and destructive thoughts that there's no place for them in your mind. It takes around six to eight weeks to firmly consolidate this change.

NEGATIVE SELF-TALK	POSITIVE THINKING
I've never done it before...	This is a chance to learn something new.
It's too complicated...	I will try from a different direction.
I'm too lazy/tired to get this done...	I'll rethink my priorities to achieve this.
There is no way this will work...	I can find a way to make this work.
No one communicates with me...	I will find a way to communicate with others.
It's too much of a major change...	I am going to give it a go.
It's not worth it...	I am worth it.

FIRE TOGETHER, WIRE TOGETHER

Have you ever been driving and realised you don't remember part of the trip? A long time ago, you taught your subconscious mind to drive the car. Now you have a kind of autopilot that allows you to think and plan, sing along to music, talk to the kids and/or have a conversation while driving. Many of your everyday actions are performed by your autopilot because you have embedded the information into your subconscious and wired your brain to perceive the world and function this way.

You can now, this very minute, continue to imprint your subconscious and rewire your brain to support your health and manage pressure differently. We are never too old to imprint or rewire new information into our brain and autopilot.

The way your brain is wired *today* is a result of your life experiences, and how you have used your brain up until now. Neuroscience and the new integrated sciences are showing that you can rewire your brain to be a servant to your needs, rather than the master of your destiny.

By dynamically interrupting your thought patterns and behaviours, and by using different perspectives to arrive at alternative solutions you will become more self-actualising and consciously aware. Doing this forces your brain to rewire and adapt.

Managing any kind of psychological or psychosocial stress, uncertainty or self-doubt is an inside-out job. When you reduce your internal pressure by thinking more helpful thoughts, you will be able to deal with external pressure in a more positive way. You will also find that you'll become more stress-resilient. Helpful thoughts, particularly pure thoughts, help you to enter and remain in your Blue Zone. It's here that you'll feel happy, curious, contented and in love with life. You'll be able to flow from one (positive) thought to another, without a need or attachment to 'fix' anything. You're purely in the moment.

'The mind is a beautiful servant or a dangerous master.'
OSHO

Your mind will lie to you if you allow it. As Mr Wong said, 'Manage your mind or it will manage you'. Your mind can be incredibly destructive. Most of your thoughts have been externally planted by your experiences in life. And sometimes they are the voice of someone else - your mother, father, siblings, teachers, or friends. Thoughts are intrinsically linked with our deepest beliefs and many of your thoughts are just trying to keep you safe. Auditing your beliefs, particularly your limiting belief system, is essential to freeing yourself to discover your full potential. We encourage you to work with trained therapists from various modalities to help you understand yourself better.

If you find you have a lot of unhelpful thoughts that take you into the dark abyss, reach out and get support. You are worth it. We have had many people tell us that after working with Journey practitioners, psychotherapists, holistic psychologists and Gestalt therapy, they feel a new sense of emotional freedom and improved self-confidence to face the challenges of life.

However, with awareness and using your brain differently, you will begin to realise: 'I am not my mind'. Changing your thoughts can lead you out of the abyss. Your new mantra:

This is only a thought, and a thought can be changed.
I am not my thoughts.

CASE STUDY

Emma

Emma's story is a classic example of how we can be hijacked by unhelpful thinking. This story also helps to understand how to catch yourself from negative thought, and audit and change these to a more helpful inner voice.

'I was running late for an appointment [classic potential Red Zone moment]. When driving through a roundabout, I took the wrong exit by mistake and didn't notice until I was a kilometre or so down the road. My autopilot was taking me on a familiar route; however that day I needed to take a different route. When I noticed the mistake, my internal dialogue was immediately destructive. "You idiot!" I told myself.

'It was untrue, I am not an idiot. The truth was, I was not paying attention, and that was how I missed the exit. I pulled to the side of the road and took a deep breath. Using my CEO to observe the situation from another perspective, I corrected my internal voice. I told myself: "It's OK. You were not paying attention. Slow down. Pay attention. Even if you are few minutes late, it's better to arrive safely".'

YOUR MOST COMMON THOUGHTS

Can you identify which are your most usual thoughts in the table below? Do your thoughts lie in the Helpful or Unhelpful column?

HELPFUL	UNHELPFUL
'I am learning and intend to try my best to do a great job of this'	'I am hopeless at this'
'I am in new territory I need to give myself some space/time to understand how to manage or process this'	'What a stupid thing to do/think'
'I am a good person doing the best I can'	'I am ugly/fat/not sexy/too old'
'I am calm and productive'	'What will people think of me' 'This always happens to me; I never have any luck etc.'
'I am happy and grateful in life'	'I am a chocaholic. I can't give up coffee/ sweets/alcohol/smoking'

BRAIN TRAINING AND WILLPOWER

By correcting your thought process in a similar way to Emma on the previous page, your CEO is activated. Remember the CEO? It's the area of your brain – the prefrontal lobe – that has the ability to perceive your thoughts and emotions as if you were the observer. Observing your thoughts from this CEO position affects your self-perception and allows your mind and brain to integrate and calm you down. Observing your thoughts from here will allow you to return to the Purple or Blue Zone. Practise is the key: audit and correct any negative or destructive thoughts as often as you can. This means paying more attention to your breathing as well as how you are thinking (more on breath work later in this chapter).

Willpower is an interesting phenomenon. We think of our willpower as something we need to force continually, however it is actually related to changing a habit or supporting ourselves to make better choices.

We need to employ willpower (focus on changing a habit) for four to eight weeks to rewire our brain. During this time, we can focus on:

- auditing our internal dialogue or inner voice
- being consciously and mindfully aware of what and how we are thinking
- talking and coaching ourselves through the challenges

While we are mindfully observing our perceptions, thoughts and emotions, the synapses in our brain are rewiring – therefore less willpower is needed as the weeks progress. We are literally rewiring our brain at every moment. By breaking down and building synapses and embedding new information into our fertile subconscious, the change will eventually register as 'normal' and less willpower will be required.

You begin to change your willpower by observing your thoughts. Do you currently think more helpful or unhelpful thoughts? Do you think your life would be changed in some way if you were to adopt more helpful thoughts? If the answer is yes, start right now. And remember to remind yourself:

How I think about what is happening to
me, is more important than what is 'actually'
happening to me.

Why?

Thoughts have meaning. Remember the lemon
visualisation earlier in this chapter.

DR KAREN ON UNHELPFUL THINKING

I have met thousands of women over time who are high achieving, amazing women, who permanently live on the edge of the Red Zone. For them, this is a normal State of Being. When I ask if they feel stressed, they reply that they feel energised. But when I take an objective peek into their day, week and month, I feel exhausted on their behalf. I see a real disconnect between their physical state and their CEO brain's assessment of how life is for them.

Understanding the consequences of unleashing the Red Zone is the start of regaining control of those stress hormones. Remember Mary's case in the last chapter? Every unhelpful or catastrophic thought Mary had produced a surge of adrenaline and elevated her normal cortisol level. Both of these reactions were designed to enable survival in humans in primitive times but, in today's world, they create a nightmare of symptoms. Disruption of the Red Zone control room by unhelpful thoughts created false life-threatening triggers which set off the cascade of falling dominos that landed Mary in Coronary Care.

Your step-by-step guide to a new way of thinking

Let's start with increasing your self-awareness of how your brain works behind the scenes. As you progress, you will start to notice your own behaviours and communication style. You'll begin to see yourself from different and new perspectives. This can be confronting because you may begin to see your unconscious behaviours and the way you interact with others. These behaviours are what other people around us see and hear.

More than 90 per cent of what you say and do throughout the day is unconscious.

By noticing more of what we do, what we think and what we say, in each moment, time slows down. You'll begin to *respond* rather than *react*. This is the beginning of the journey to increase your ability to activate the CEO brain. The CEO brain has the ability to self-observe and help you manage the monkey brain.

Unpacking a little more about the brain can give some reference point in learning how to notice your reaction and behaviours. It will help you understand which part of your brain is dominant under pressure.

UNDERSTANDING THE LIMBIC/MONKEY BRAIN

We exhibit the four Fs
when we are under too much pressure:

FIGHT:
our limbic/monkey brain takes over

FLIGHT:
our limbic/monkey brain takes over

FREEZE:
our limbic/monkey brain and prefrontal lobe are both activated

FAINT:
our systems overload and we lose consciousness

The monkey brain can be quite black and white. It is constantly judging if you are safe or unsafe. It can only see right or wrong because it does not have a global perspective to see any variation or grey areas. Your monkey brain will try to manipulate every situation to ensure your safety. However the amygdala (emotional sensor) is capable of hijacking your brain. When this happens, you may react and behave inappropriately or feel a sense of panic because you are blinded by a 'perception' of danger.

The monkey brain has strong, subconscious views and a territorial motor. In times of pressure, a person moves to a more reactive state and can sometimes find themselves playing controlling games (more on these games later in this chapter).

STUCK IN THE MIDDLE – ARE YOU?

The monkey brain also has a great need to be right, which was important for the survival of our ancient ancestors. Have you ever experienced someone being totally unreasonable about a matter, and regardless of how you approach the subject they still refuse to shift their perspective? Has this ever happened to you, where you're stuck in 'the principle'?

In the Red Zone, the monkey brain struggles to see other perspectives and can hold deep resentment and hostility. At worst, it can seek revenge.

We know from science that hostility and resentment is debilitating for heart health and your DNA via epigenetic changes, and is responsible for shortening telomeres (the end caps on your chromosomes that define our genetic health). Negative emotions such as anger, frustration, greed, self-righteousness and resentment produce bio-chemicals that drive the hormone cortisol.

The monkey brain in full flight can also lead you to manipulate others so they will agree to be on your side (the ancient game of 'safety in numbers'). This can play out as a disagreement that causes division between family members, colleagues or friends. Some agree with one person and some agree with the other, and people become fixated on who is right. This can escalate and cause the complete breakdown of a team or family unit. Sound familiar?

How to understand the 'new' brain

You can help yourself to move to and stay in the Purple and Blue Zones by noticing your behaviours and communication styles. The art of self-observation helps you to understand which part of your brain you are operating from: the limbic monkey, or the prefrontal CEO.

Knowing you are in 'fear' mode, or noticing that others around are, can help you to understand different perspectives and train your brain differently. The more you train yourself to use the evolved parts of the brain, rather than the monkey when you are under pressure, the better your response to pressure becomes. These parts of your brain are known as the 'new' brain, involving the neocortex, the social brain, and the prefrontal lobe. Actively recruiting these parts of your brain in daily life can help a lot.

THE PREFRONTAL CORTEX (YOUR CEO)

Remember, the prefrontal cortex is the CEO of your brain and the basis of your incredible intelligence. We have already established that the CEO has the ability to perceive your thoughts and emotions as if you were the observer.

Further, this part of your brain, along with the essential 'social part' also allows you to sense and imagine another person's thoughts, feelings and memories. This insight can allow you to perceive a more global perspective and various points of view, an important skill that changes how you understand yourself and how you see the world.

When you move into the CEO of your brain, you can observe and better understand the nature of the monkey brain. Neuroscience believes that it is from the CEO brain that humans are able to moderate and manage the reactivity of the monkey brain. This is thought to be because the CEO brain allows you to self-actualise and to see things more globally. In conjunction with the neocortex, it also offers you a great deal of creative solutions, emotional intelligence and a conscious awareness that allows you to see people from different perspectives.

Rather than blaming others for their controlling behaviour and B.A.D communication style (see page 320 for more on B.A.D communication), you could instead view them as a victim of their unmanaged monkey brain.

Don't take it personally. Instead, think: 'Oh goodness, you poor thing. The monkey has you by the tail and you are definitely not yourself right now.' This way you are objectifying and rationalising someone else's behaviour. Moving deeper, you may be able to see another person's behaviour as a latent reaction to a deep emotional wound, not enough sleep, or ongoing debilitating pressures. This is a particular skill of the CEO brain.

When operating from these newer parts of your brain, you will have emotional intelligence and understand social consequences. You will be able to form deep and meaningful relationships with other humans in your life.

Your CEO, neocortex and social brain allows you to use thoughts, feelings and memories in new and helpful ways. You have the ability to go beyond being sad or being angry; you can recognise that your feelings are not the totality of who you are. By naming your emotions you can learn how to understand them, making your inner world less scary.

With support from a trained professional, these parts of your brain can help you understand and reappraise past hurts and emotional wounds. You will also learn how to manage your thoughts and emotions through a wider mental funnel.

This type of emotional therapy is often called exposure therapy. Neuroscience research shows we are able to desensitise our amygdala and are therefore no longer able to be hijacked into an emotional response.

When trained, the CEO has the ability to moderate the monkey brain impulses. It is able to negotiate calmly and fairly. It understands the higher levels of emotion, such as forgiveness, compassion, empathy and justice for all.

The CEO needs strong blood flow and lots of conscious stimulation. A very active prefrontal lobe will result in a calm, intuitive, rational, creative and productive person. Training this part of your brain should be a priority.

When Nelson Mandela tried to unite the people of South Africa following the end of apartheid, his approach was a demonstration of upper and CEO brain genius.

He coached the captain of South Africa's national rugby team, the Springboks, to inspire his team to win the World Cup. He also arranged for the team, before they played in the World Cup, to travel around the country and coach children in Black communities.

This inspired hope across the country. When the Springboks played in the World Cup, all South Africans - regardless of colour - had something in common; they wanted their country's team to win.

Indeed, the Springboks did go on to win the Cup and this first step built a tiny bridge to begin the long and difficult journey of unifying a country divided by apartheid. This particular example of leadership is considered to be a legendary initiative by Mr Mandela and is brilliant evidence of his highly developed CEO brain pathways.

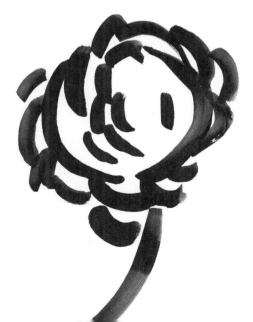

YOUR ACTION PLAN

How to manage stress on a day-to-day basis

Psychological stress is managed from the inside out, rather than the outside in. Prioritising your tasks and managing them effectively is important, as is the effective use of communication and time. However, it is the internal influences that have the greatest effect on our stress levels.

Throughout the day you will need to use your internal dialogue and internal awareness to self-coach through the rough patches. The following concepts can help train your upper brain to navigate life and see the experiences you encounter with more acceptance and compassion:

Mindfulness
Diaphragmatic breathing
Managing the monkey

Mindfulness

Mindfulness is awareness that arises through paying attention, on purpose, in the present moment, non-judgementally, in the service of self-understanding and wisdom.

JON KABAT-ZINN

We are all living in a preconditioned illusion. Due to this conditioned perspective, we may be missing the magnificent truth of who we are; indescribable, intelligent consciousness with unlimited potential.

The practice of mindfulness is an upper-brain activity. When you practice this way of perceiving the world, noticing your thoughts and feelings, you activate your CEO brain and become more conscious of your conditioned, perceptive lenses.

One of the aspects of mindfulness is understanding the relationship between your physical and mental self.

Mindfulness is the lens through which we observe our inner and outer worlds, simply being open and curious, flexible and willing to see different perspectives without criticism and judgment. The simplest explanation is to be in the moment wherever you are; when you are in the yoga class, be in the yoga class; when you are thinking and planning, do this; when you are with your children and loved ones, be present with your children and loved ones.

Mindfulness is key to our ability to manage uncertainty, self-doubt and pressure, particularly internal pressure. This helps us to activate our action plan for managing a stressful life.

BACK TO THE FUTURE

With our current understanding of physics, it is not possible for you to take your body back in time to last week, last year or 20 years ago. Nor is it possible to take your body forward in time. Your body is always here, in this moment. If you pay attention to each moment and open your senses to what you smell, see, and hear, you will feel the present, and within this, notice your presence. Your breath reminds you of this simple realisation, with each breath in and out, you will notice this moment in time. This is mindfulness in action.

Non mindfulness is when the mind takes over. The mind is by nature a time traveller. If your mind travels to the past it may wonder: 'I could have'; 'I should have', 'if only'; and may have regrets.

If your mind travels to the future, it moves into pure speculation. Some people may catastrophise and imagine all sorts of 'what if' scenarios, worrying about situations that may never happen. Your mind will also create expectations about how things *should* look, and play this out. Any deviation from this imagined, idealised future will result in disappointment, created by the invention of your own speculation.

While it is necessary to think and make plans, doing so with a mindful approach is key. Setting yourself up for 'expectation failure' is a common human flaw.

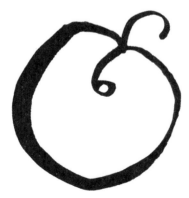

CASE STUDY

Sarah

Sarah is a caregiver for her disabled son and also runs a busy business from her home. She wasn't sleeping or eating properly and noticed that more often than not her day started by warming up with several cups of coffee and cooling down with at least a half bottle of wine. She was, she realised, exhausted.

She decided to take some time out and book a healthy holiday. She did her research, made the booking and waited patiently. She daydreamed of the idealised situation she so desperately needed. She had a mental picture in her mind of exactly how her room and how the place should be; this was her imagined perfect setting, and her heart was set on it.

The day came, and she arrived at the destination. The setting was not exactly how she had imagined it and she became incredibly upset and disappointed. She cried to herself because the room was all wrong. It was facing the wrong direction and it was the wrong colour. She had a neighbour who she just knew would be noisy. She had planned this holiday for months and now it was all ruined. Her thoughts became unhelpful. Her monkey was yelling and she had been pushed in the Red Zone. She thought: 'How could this happen to me? It's not fair. I work so hard and I needed this to be perfect. And it's not.'

In her totally depleted state, Sarah was inconsolable. Even though the team at the destination bent over backwards to make her feel comfortable, all she could see was what was wrong with the room. Because it did not match the picture in her mind that she had imagined, she was now devastated.

Luckily, the team understood Sarah's depleted state, and, with empathy and compassion gained her trust. After a few days, when Sarah stopped 'living in her head' and began to look around with mindfulness, she realised that this place was perfect for what she needed. The natural surroundings had somehow soothed her soul, the wildlife delighted her and the food was nourishing and delicious. Her neighbour turned out to be a wonderful person, who Sarah now knew would become a life friend. She realised her room was cosy and comfortable; although it was not what she'd imagined, she realised it was the ideal space to allow her to rest and recover. In fact, she realised that this destination was actually perfect, and surprisingly better than what she had imagined for herself.

Sarah's story is a reminder that sometimes you don't always get what you want. Yet, if you ask yourself: 'Where is the good in this situation?', it may be just what you need. Life presents constant challenges; it's how you think about what is happening that will make the most difference.

A positive mindful frame on any situation can improve your perception of whatever you are facing and help you self-regulate where you need to be: Purple Flow or the Blue Zone.

The power of the breath

The so-called Yi (the mind) is the horse of the breath.
When moving or stopping, they follow each other.

T'AI HSI CHING CHU, *THE EMBRYONIC BREATH CANON*

From the moment you take your first breath until the moment you take your last, this essential element for life has enormous influence on your mind and body. When observed, your breath can give focus to the mind, slow your heart rate, reduce blood pressure and bring internal quiet and stillness into focus.

The ancient and traditional healing systems, such as Ayurveda (from which yoga is derived), have known the significance of the breath and its patterns for centuries.

Yoga is the home of focused breathing. It teaches you to breathe in challenging poses and this learning can be transferred to your daily life. Learning to notice and focus on your breathing whenever you feel self-doubt, pressured, or notice your body's stress response, you can change your physiology by changing the depth, rhythm and pace of your breathing.

On a physical level, research shows that diaphragmatic breathing - when each breath takes the diaphragm through its full range of motion - moves you out of the Red Zone. Paying attention to, and changing, your breathing pattern is a powerful ally in a fast-paced busy life. Breath is free and is constantly with you; you simply need to remember and pay attention.

On a consciousness level, breath connects every one of us. Every intake of breath is an acceptance of life - you breathe in a gas that is given off by plants and trees. Every time you breathe out, you're letting go, and the gas you exhale is essential for the life of plants and trees. In this simple way, we are all connected.

This cycle of giving and receiving has been present for centuries and will continue long after your lifetime. Yet many of us can go through life, lost in thought, disconnected from the essence of who we are.

The practice of mindfulness and meditation teaches you to pay attention to the messages your body is sending. Noticing you are shallow breathing and then actively changing to deep, belly breathing will help you calm down and move to parts of your brain that have more solutions and a better decision-making ability.

Qi Gong, Pilates and yoga are some of the activities you can engage in to learn greater breath control.

STRAW BREATHING

Imagine you have a straw in your mouth. Form your lips into the shape they would take if you were holding the straw. Now draw air through the imaginary straw all the way to your belly. Hold your breath in for a moment until you feel the need to breathe out. Exhale through the imaginary straw and hold the breath out until you feel the need to breathe in. Repeat this for 3-4 breath cycles.

Do you notice that your mind is focused on your breath? This can be used as a circuit breaker for a busy mind, particularly in times of extreme pressure.

DAY-TO-DAY BREATHING

1   Begin every day by being aware of your breath.

2   Being aware of your breath will give you focus. Set an intention for your day – be mindful to pay attention to your breath each moment and remind yourself to regulate your breathing whenever you become challenged or busy.

3   Throughout your day, notice your breathing. A faster pace of breath will be required in a spin class, a slower deeper pace in a massage.

4   A quiet walk will allow you to notice your breathing while walking in nature. You may notice how much is missed when you walk and talk with others. Try to take walks on your own and reflect on how beautiful it is to be in nature. Be silent and listen to the rhythm of your own breathing. Feel gratitude or awareness of being alive on a brand-new day.

5   You can practise your breathing wherever you are, whatever you are doing. This is the beauty and simplicity of the breath. Simply pay more attention to your breathing in different situations in life.

6   In challenging moments, try to deepen your breathing and slow its pace. If you wake in the middle of the night, rather than thinking, planning and organising, bring your awareness to focus on deep belly breathing. This induces the body to relax. With the mind engaged on the breath you will naturally fall back asleep.

Our health and wellbeing are dependent on many elements; however, breath is the unsung hero. Learning how to relax is as simple as breathing in and breathing out. Why not practise right now?

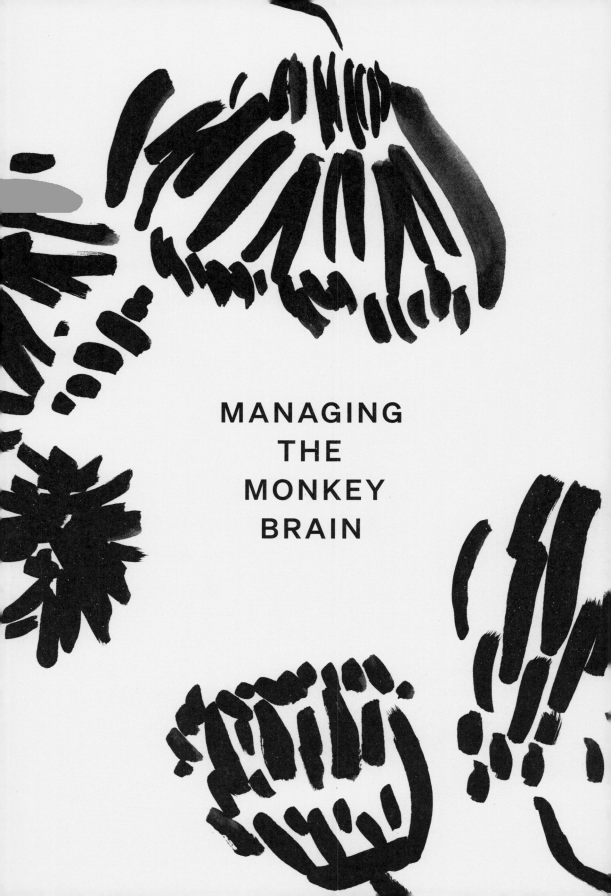

MANAGING
THE
MONKEY
BRAIN

1.
Taming the monkey

These steps, in this order, will help you to calm yourself and support your ability to respond to situations rather than react. This includes times when you're feeling impatient, intolerant, frustrated, angry, overwhelmed, sad, anxious or panicky. Find additional strategies for exiting the Red Zone on page 271.

STEP ONE

Observe what you are feeling and name the emotion. For example: 'I am feeling angry at the moment'. The monkey brain does not know the name of our emotion, but the CEO does know the name. This helps to recruit our upper brain to moderate and manage the monkey.

STEP TWO

Take a deep breath. Continue to focus on your breath. Use the straw breath routine (outlined on page 312) or diaphragmatic breathing. Make every effort to slow your breathing.

STEP THREE

Observe your thinking and focus on helpful thoughts.

STEP FOUR

Slow your speaking and listen closely to what you are saying.

STEP FIVE

Repeat Steps One to Four until you feel calm and centred.

2.

Manage your mind: an exercise

Imagine your mind is a monkey that sits on your shoulder, whispering into your ear every moment of every day. Your job is to listen and pay attention to what the monkey is saying (particularly in times of pressure). You will analyse something as a 'helpful or unhelpful' thought. If the thought is unhelpful, we simply say to the monkey: 'That's unhelpful. Do you have a helpful thought?'.

Whilst this sounds strange, what this practice allows you to do is see that an aspect of your thoughts comes from an objectified source, one that is separate to you. This gives you the power to change the thought in real time. This offers your internal voice an opportunity to think more positively and objectively.

After a while of practising this, when you hear unhelpful thoughts you will simply acknowledge: 'That's the monkey, not me.'

It works, try it!

3.

Are you being too controlling? The games we all play

Control is held in great esteem by the monkey brain. Feeling in control can often give you a sense of power and help you feel that you are safe. However, almost every one of us has very little control of what happens in life – which is why many people cling to a sinking life raft, struggling to gain more and more control. Ultimately, it just slips through your fingers.

When in the Red Zone, you may find that you unconsciously try to gain control of situations and others. To do this, four controlling behaviours come into play. These are not in any order – whatever has worked for you for most of your life will be the one that you will try first.

1. THE NICE GAME
2. THE NASTY GAME
3. THE MOODY GAME
4. THE VICTIM GAME

1. THE NICE GAME

Have you ever met or dealt with someone who is extraordinarily nice? They compliment you, tell you everything you want to hear, then ask you to do something you are not keen to do. All the time they have been talking, you get the feeling that they have an agenda. It feels like a sales pitch; they want you to do something for them. It may feel difficult to say no because they are 'just so nice'. Of course, the nice game is the 'nicest' of the four games. But let's not sugarcoat it – it's manipulation. Often when you do not come around to their way of thinking or do what they are asking, they will quickly flip into another game.

2. THE NASTY GAME

As the name suggests, this is when someone is arrogant, rude, aggressive, threatening, or bullying – either loudly or subversively. This is the game of threat, survival of the fittest. Most people who exhibit this kind of behaviour have at some point experienced an emotional wound, or they are emotionally insecure. Their behaviour is to shield you (and themselves) from seeing their truth. This game in full flight can be one of the most frightening and intensive you'll witness or experience. Sometimes the game can flip from nice to nasty, and you'll see the true colours of a person emerge.

3. THE MOODY GAME

Typified by monosyllabic answers and cold shoulder tactics, this game is to cut off any communication in the supreme effort to control the situation. This is the one we often play with friends and family. The truth is, we do not do this to improve communication, we do it to be noticed and to try to regain the front-foot position in whatever altercation is presenting. Stuck in hurt, we refuse to forgive or move from the position of 'it's the principle' in a supreme effort of one upmanship.

4. THE VICTIM GAME

We could write another book on this game; it is so prevalent in society. This is where we want others to feel sorry for us, because we may or may not have faced some difficulty or adversity. This is actually one of the most controlling of all the games. There is a triad that plays out here of victim, persecutor and rescuer. Interestingly, each have an identity associated with this game and as a result, have a stake in the game. Sometimes a rescuer does not want the victim to heal because they will then have no one to rescue. This game is our default program for times when challenges are overwhelming. The game is also perhaps needed when our life is threatened and a member of the tribe risks their life to save us.

In a perfect world, when someone needs support (the victim) there is support from others (the rescuer) until the victim has recovered physically or emotionally from an event. However, some victims get stuck and can't shake the need to be the victim. The tricky part is that it doesn't matter how many people come to their aid, they are the only ones who can rescue themselves.

When stuck, a victim mentality imagines that the world and everyone else is more powerful than themselves. Believing themselves to be helpless in their circumstance, they may continue to disempower themselves by staying stuck in their story and therefore not realise their potential. Sometimes this has been wired into their brain by well-meaning parents or other influences that have raised a child to believe this is the best they can be.

There are true victims in life. These are people who live life with deep scars after facing some horrific event or those who are truly disabled. There are also those who have faced the unthinkable and who have somehow brushed themselves off and become a shining light of humanity, sharing their learnings with the world.

It is easy to be swept away by some overwhelming feeling, so it's helpful to remember that any stressful feeling is like a compassionate alarm clock that says, 'You're caught in the dream.' Depression, pain, and fear are gifts that say, 'Sweetheart, take a look at your thinking right now. You're living in a story that isn't true for you.'

BYRON KATIE

LOVING WHAT IS: FOUR QUESTIONS THAT CAN CHANGE YOUR LIFE

HOW SELF-AWARE ARE YOU?

Often when we're in the Red Zone we are not self-aware, because the monkey brain is not self-aware. We may not notice the games we play, or the style of communication we adopt.

When you feel stressed, try to notice and pay attention to these games and communication styles in yourself, and in others. Doing this recruits the CEO brain, which helps you to regain internal control and return to the Purple and Blue Zones. By taking stock or your actions and your reactions, you're approaching a situation – personal or professionally – with your very best intentions and ability.

When in the Red Zone our communication often disintegrates and you may have a tendency to use a BAD form of communication.

WHAT IS B.A.D COMMUNICATION?
B: Blaming someone or something for what has happened or is about to happen
A: Attacking anyone or anything. You may feel justified to take matters into your own hands
D: Defending your own actions and/or pointing the finger of blame elsewhere

When you're in the Red Zone you have a great need to be right. This is thought to be one of our ancient survival tactics, as making the right decision could often mean life or death. Today, it is usually played out by being very rigid in a viewpoint or holding on to 'the principle'.

Give me principle over logic anytime.

DAME MAGGIE SMITH

AS LADY VIOLET CRAWLEY, *DOWNTON ABBEY*

Five additional strategies for stress resilience

1   Keep your internal battery charged
2   Spend more time in the Blue Zone
3   Practice Qi Gong
4   Change gears
5   Press pause

Energy is the body's currency. Energy production is not just about getting fuel from food. It's also important to preserve our energy by spending sufficient amounts of quality time in the Blue Zone.

As discussed in Chapter 6 and 7, just like your mobile phone needs to be charged every night in order to function, so does your body. Charging your mobile phone is non-negotiable, the phone simply won't function unless you charge it. Guess what, our body is the same. Spending time in the Blue Zone is the equivalent of charging your body to heal, rest, recover and is non-negotiable to the body. We are designed to spend a significant amount of time in the Blue Zone and a good night's sleep is simply not enough. Prioritising spending time in the Blue Zone will activate the following 10 essential functions within your body (there are many more):

✓   Reduce your resting brain state, mentioned in Chapter 7
✓   Repair and renew all cells in your body, including heart and brain cells
✓   Improve your immune system to help ward off colds, flus and viruses as well as help heal any medical diagnosis
✓   Reduce inflammation in the body
✓   Provide the ideal environment for a healthy, diverse gut microbiome
✓   Improve sleep quality
✓   Improve digestion and heal gut inflammation
✓   Balance hormones
✓   Reduce resting heart rate and blood pressure
✓   Keep a healthy gene expression and reduce negative gene activity

Nervous system recharge and energy use

BLUE ZONE

Energy and healing is recharged - increasing Qi boosts the recharging. Entering the Blue Zone and Qi are explained later in this chapter.

PURPLE ZONE

We use energy in the Purple Flow Zone although it is a slow burn. Rather than feeling exhausted at the end of our day, we feel satisfied and find it easy to relax.

RED ZONE

Energy is burned quickly which causes energy levels to be depleted. Exhaustion sets in and we often find it difficult to relax. We can feel wired and very tired.

The ideas below will help you boost your stress resilience. Using this as a way of life will help prevent you depleting your energy stores, working with your body rather than against it. It is essential that you learn how to manage your bodies non-negotiable needs.

By managing your internal pressure, you will have the ability to be in your Purple Flow Zone when you need to get things done and then return to the Blue Zone to build and maintain your internal battery life. The following table will help you navigate, conserve and recharge your energy and Qi.

STAGE ONE

Prediction

STAGE TWO

Manage pressure in the moment

STAGE THREE

Recovery

HOW TO NAVIGATE, CONSERVE AND RECHARGE

	ASK YOURSELF	YOUR ANSWER
STRESS RESILIENCE STAGE ONE		
PREDICTION	'Will there be some challenges ahead that are going to put pressure on me?' 'What can I do now to prepare myself to manage these future pressures?'	Ensure I have enough energy in reserve by spending more time in the Blue Zone and building my Qi.
STRESS RESILIENCE STAGE TWO		
HOW TO MANAGE PRESSURE IN THE MOMENT	'How can I deal with difficult and challenging situations in the most calm and effective manner as possible?'	Follow the stress management pyramid earlier in the chapter (see page 281). · Before you respond to somebody, or a task (such as an email), take a pause · Listen and evaluate before replying (in person or via email) · Accept what is and what you cannot change
STRESS RESILIENCE STAGE THREE		
RECOVERY	'When I have been under pressure, what do I need to do to process and manage what just happened?' 'How can I give myself and my body the time to recover from this onslaught of pressure?'	'I need to restore my energy levels by spending time in the Blue Zone and cultivating my Qi.'

STRATEGIES

- Prioritise sleep
- 3-4 alcohol free days per week
- Eat clean nutritious food
- Minimise daily caffeine intake from all sources

- Acupuncture
- Reduce social commitments
- Get some gentle exercise
- Think positively about your ability to deal with any situation that may arise

- Turn unhelpful thoughts into helpful thoughts
- Be your own internal coach
- Prioritise diaphragmatic breathing throughout your day
- Have early nights as often as possible
- Drink plenty of water

- Eat well
- Have regular massages
- Enjoy hot baths with Epsom salts
- Meditate (mornings are best)
- Take time to do nothing

- Diaphragmatic breathing - this is the only manual override that will move you from the Red Zone to the Blue Zone. (Other natural body functions are laughing, sighing and yawning.)
- Cuddle a loved one
- Creative cooking: forget the meal planning. Try a new recipe
- Try pottery, painting, knitting or sewing
- Pick up a pen and do some creative writing or journalling
- Daily meditation and visualisation
- Restorative yoga
- Watch a sunset
- Spend some time in nature

- Take a bath
- Visit a waterfall
- Float in water (the pool, ocean or even bathtub)
- Watch the clouds
- Enjoy a picnic in the park
- Take a nap under an umbrella in the fresh air
- Read a book (avoid anything too 'thrilling')
- Watch a movie (a comedy rather than a Whodunnit!)
- Reduce alcohol consumption

RECOVERY

As has been mentioned many times earlier in this book, spending time in the Blue Zone is where your essential recovery happens. How each person finds their way into their Blue Zone state is different. Please be mindful that entering this zone can't involve alcohol or non-prescription drugs, so having a glass of something to chill out is not for this occasion. Explore these ideas to support you to relax and recover or find your own way. Remember blue zoning is a non-active state. It is about allowing your mind to settle.

No matter what you choose, include diaphragmatic breathing and helpful thoughts. This is all about making and taking time for you. Finding your own pathway is an essential step into your personal recovery mode.

Creativity: Painting, drawing, photography, creative writing, pottery, colouring in, calligraphy and anything along these lines that allows you to get lost in the moment, where your breathing is slow and you are loving what you are doing.

Nature: Spending time outdoors is quite literally a salve to the nervous system so bathing in nature whilst not doing much is a great way to relax. Lying watching the clouds, sitting on the beach, floating in water, picnic somewhere with a view, sitting in a hot springs, watch the sunrise/sunset, watch and listen to the rain, night gazing at the moon and stars, simply close your eyes and open all your other senses. Sit on the grass, dig your feet into sand.

Connection: Hugging and cuddling loved ones, connect to your breath, relax with your animals, marvel at natural scenes and celebrate the awe of nature, laughing with friends, living in the moment.

Spa treatments: Acupuncture (it's a body hack into the Blue Zone), body scrubs and wraps, relaxing facials and massages (the ones that make you dribble and drool), an aromatic restorative bath, a sauna or steam room.

THE POWER OF QI

Ancient Eastern philosophy recognised thousands of years ago that we are more than just cells and bones; we are also an energetic system. This is compatible with Western medicine's evolution that understands we are essentially the product of protons, neutrons and electrons and all the space in between.

In Chinese medicine, the ancients referred to the meridian system (energy channels). This is the focus of acupuncture, as the metal needles assist in the electrical transfer of Qi (pronounced chi) through our meridians. A Traditional Chinese Medicine Practitioner (TCM) will treat according to the flow of Qi or where Qi may be 'stuck' or not flowing in the body.

However, Qi in Chinese medicine also comes from Jing (primordial essence, the Qi we inherit from our parents and ancestors) and Shen (spirit energy, our individual Qi). The Qi flows though meridians and concentrates into dantians, which play a similar role to the chakras and vary in number according to the system.

The ancient practice of Qi Gong (similar to the movement of tai chi) can be simply described as a moving meditation, although it has a much deeper philosophy around energy and is derived from Chinese Medicine. Most practitioners of this ancient, powerful, traditional healing system practice Qi Gong movements to harness their own Qi for treating their patients.

The meaning of Qi Gong is, quite simply, moving energy around. This is more simplistic than the true translation. However, we do not have words in the English language to describe the essence of the true meaning. When practiced with the movements, it looks like tai chi and, like most martial arts, is focused on mindfulness practice. There are three parts: breath, connection and awareness to the moment. Slow deliberate movements are designed to open the meridian channels to allow Qi to flow.

According to the ancient Chinese masters, everything in nature has Qi: the trees, ground, ocean, sky and all creatures. Humans have Qi; however the practice of Qi Gong allows us to continuously recharge our main Qi storage area in the lower abdomen.

WHERE IS YOUR QI?

You can find your 'Qi storage area' quite easily. Place three fingers below your navel. About one-third of the way inside you is a place referred to as the dantian. This is one of the main storage areas for our Qi. (There are others, but for simplicity we are just focusing on this one.) Many people have depleted their Qi and therefore have little charge to their energy system. These people often walk around exhausted and have no idea how to replenish their energy.

We often use this analogy to explain Qi: have you ever worked in the office all day and felt physically exhausted when you stand up to leave? How can this be when you have burned almost no calories at all?

What you have used up is your Qi. Your energy, literally your life force, is drained.

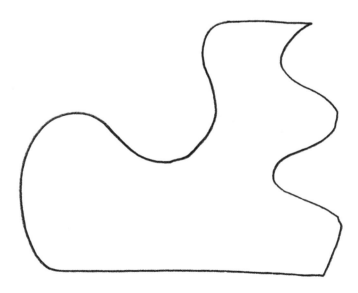

QI AND THE CITY

Sharon says: 'I was reminded of how cities can drain you of Qi when I was on a trip to New York in 2015. A few days after arriving, I felt exhausted, surrounded by so many people bustling about. There was so much concrete and electromagnetic energy. I remember looking out the apartment window at all the buildings stacked together and thinking that if I had X-ray eyes I'd see a city made up of millions and millions of wires filled with electricity and Wi-Fi. All this, surrounding millions of humans stacked on top of one another. We now know for sure; this way of living has an impact on human health.

'Although I loved exploring such a vibrant city and spending time with dear friends, I tried to make it to Central Park every day to recharge, as being in nature is a great way to restore Qi. However, sadly after three weeks I became really ill and ended up with bronchitis – something I had never had before. By the time I returned home my body was in such a depleted state it needed serious restoration. It took a couple of months to fully recover.'

HOW TO RESTORE YOUR QI

Your Qi energy cannot be restored effectively by exercise and food alone. Qi is quickly diminished by too much thinking, planning and doing. Like a candle flame burning in a draught, the wax drips and the candle burns unevenly.

Without replenishing it, over time your Qi will become depleted. Qi restoration comes from connection to our self, the earth, the universe and each other. Traditional Chinese Medicine practitioners can advise you how to improve your Qi and identify the kind of Qi you are lacking.

HOW TO SAVE AND RESTORE YOUR QI

Restoring

Every day, find some time in nature and practise being present with your body. Feel your feet on the ground, your breath moving in and out from your belly. Sense what is in the moment: smells, sound, touch and sight. You may like to visualise growing roots from your feet into the ground below you, and with every breath in draw energy and vitality from the earth itself into your dantian. Just doing this mindful exercise for even 5-10 minutes each day, without the movements, is a lovely way to connect to yourself and nature, naturally recharging your Qi.

Saving

As life goes on, whenever you feel overwhelmed, confused or challenged, take a moment to centre yourself and use some internal positive coaching. Speak to yourself kindly and with compassion – this is an important step in supporting yourself to learn how to effectively navigate internal and external pressure.

Acknowledge to yourself when you are overwhelmed. Use a calm inner voice filled with helpful thoughts. This may be: 'Okay, I am in new territory here, I am not sure what to do or where to go with this. I will just remind myself to focus on my breathing and take baby steps. I will learn, one step at a time, what needs to happen. With each step this will be one less thing I need to learn in the future.'

If you feel comfortable, you may want to share these moments with others in your life simply telling them: 'I feel uncertain right now, and I need some time to process and manage my internal world to find the next step forward. Thank you for your patience with me. I just need some time to work this out.'

This can be a very powerful way to help your children. The words: 'Mummy is processing what has just happened', can give both parties time to absorb and reflect. These words can help your child understand that even parents need some time to figure things out. This helps them to emulate your emotional world and way of communicating. It can encourage them – and you – to positively self-coach.

If you want to know what your thoughts were like in the past, feel your body. If you want to know what your body will feel like in the future, look at your thoughts today.

CHANGING GEARS

It's important to recognise that we all play different roles in life. For example, Sharon is a professional speaker, wellness consultant, stress resilience mentor and facilitator of Equine Assisted Learning in her working life. At home, she is mother, grandmother, sister, auntie, friend and horse rider. Karen is a doctor at work and at home she's a gardener, mother, daughter, sister, friend, and lover of travelling and new languages. Moving from one role to the other means we all need to change gears.

Imagine driving down the highway at 120km an hour. Now take the exit ramp. You will need to slow down to be able to navigate the smaller streets, stop lights, pedestrians and so on. Otherwise, you will most likely do some damage.

The same applies in daily life. We need to change gears depending on the situation. If you're at work and going into a meeting, you may need to 'travel' at a different speed than if you were giving a presentation.

The same applies at home. Your family does not want the CEO/professional/worker. Think of the front door as the divider between the 'worker you' and the 'real you'. Our friends and family want their loved one to walk through the door and engage in a relationship that is respectful, and full of love and trust.

If you do work at home, do something to try to separate your two lives: the worker you and the real you. Keep the boundary and watch how things evolve. It may help to have an office in a separate room which has a door that shuts or a defined workspace with a plant divider. Aim to set office hours so that you're not checking emails when it's family time; or take a walk or even just go into your garden or outside space at the end of the day as part of your 'commute'. The sanctuary of the home is best shielded from outside challenges whenever possible, so that it remains a space for you to rest and revive. (See Chapter 6 for advice on how to develop healthy boundaries).

Following a traumatic experience, often many people say that during the trauma, all they could think about was wanting their family and friends to know how much they love them. When we strip it all back, the most precious things in our life have nothing to do with what we own. Yet when we get stressed and tired, we hurt the people we love the most because we are not managing our awareness and being mindful of each individual situation.

PRESSING PAUSE

Put life on hold by taking a walk in nature, doing a short meditation, running a bath, fully inhaling with a deep breath. It is simply something you can do as you change gears and can be used both personally and professionally to clear your mind and activate your prefrontal lobe.

Try the following visualisation. It takes just 15 seconds.

Close your eyes. Focus on your breath coming into your belly. Now focus on your mind. You are on a swing. You may be in the country or by the beach. You can be your current age, or older, or younger. As you imagine yourself on the swing, envisage the movements you would need your body to make in order to get the swing to move until it's at a height you feel comfortable with. Now, stretch your arms and legs and let the swing move you. Feel the air blowing through your hair.

Swing back and forth for several cycles. Now open your eyes.
Simple, isn't it? How do you feel? Your monkey brain can't do this visualisation – only your upper brain can visualise such a scenario. (Note: you can be fishing, watching the sun set, lying in a hammock – anything you like. The point is to close your eyes and imagine a positive scene.)

This is a great visualisation to do prior to an event – before you give a presentation; before you go into an important meeting; before a first date; or when you drive into your driveway before you enter your home.

Mindfulness is a practice of paying attention with a sense of openness, curiosity and acceptance to whatever is arising in the present moment.

DR DANIEL FRIEDLAND

Time to rest.

Welcome to Pillar Four

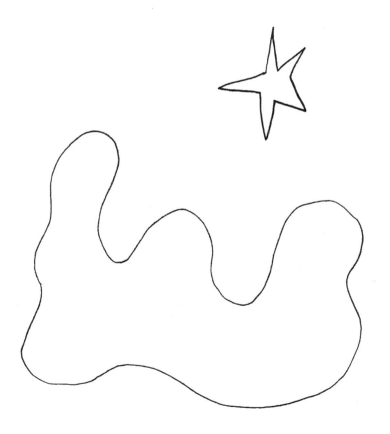

9.
SLEEP

Nothing is permanent, this too will pass.

BUDDHA

One of the most important pillars of wellness is quality sleep. This essential part of everyday life is as important as food, and needs to be a priority if you want to thrive. If you're in a Depleted or Surviving state and you're experiencing poor-quality sleep, addressing this should be one of the first steps towards whole health. Every adult requires at least seven to eight hours of sleep every 24 hours, and teenagers need even more. Restorative sleep is best achieved by following the body's natural circadian rhythm. Ironically, you also need to have enough energy to sleep.

What is a good night's sleep?

GOOD-QUALITY SLEEP IS DEFINED AS:

- Going to bed and falling asleep within 15 minutes of your head touching the pillow.

- Sleeping deeply for seven to eight hours and waking naturally without an alarm, feeling refreshed.

- If you wake once or twice through the night to go to the bathroom, this is still considered fine if you're able to go straight back to sleep.

HOW TO GET YOUR BODY CLOCK TICKING ON TIME

Humans are hardwired to sleep when it's dark and to be productive when the sun shines. But the microscopic world within also ticks to its own biological rhythm. Your innate body clock is accurate to the second.

Your bio-clock that has been thoroughly studied is the one responsible for the opening hours of the 'Factory of Happiness', better known in medical circles as the 'Serotonin Production Factory'. This essential nervous system hormone buffers you through bad times and helps you appreciate the good times in life.

This factory is open for business during a particular part of the normal sleep cycle called Deep Sleep. To support this nervous system hormone you need to spend an appropriate amount of time in Deep Sleep. The ironic twist is that the sleep hormone melatonin is built from recycled serotonin. These two hormones are intimately linked – when one is disrupted the other will also fail to deliver. You can begin to understand how important sleep is to your ability to cultivate happiness. On a typical night when sleep comes easily, you should enter Deep Sleep two to three times.

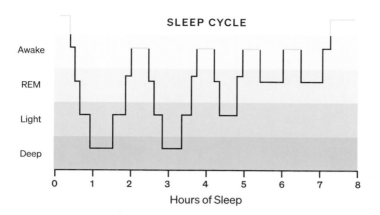

WHAT DOES DEEP SLEEP FEEL LIKE?

Imagine the following: a family arrives home, a sleeping toddler in their arms. The young child has its nappy changed and then is put into bed without so much as a yawn – so completely and utterly deep is the sleep for this child. Welcome to Deep Sleep, where restorative work happens, and happiness begins. It's why we have the saying 'sleeping like a baby'.

How many times in a week do you wake up and truly say: 'Yes, I got a great night's sleep last night'? Most likely you got less than you needed, and your sleep habits need tweaking to avoid the increased risk of health challenges developing.

Chronically disrupted sleep doubles the risk of dying from just about everything! Let's look at what happens when you don't get a quality eight hours sleep a night. There is an increased risk of the following medical diseases:

- Heart disease and stroke
- Type 2 diabetes
- Cancer
- Kidney disease
- Clinical depression
- Anxiety and panic attacks

You will feel so good after a great night's rest, it's probably enough motivation to look at putting into action the solutions for better sleep.

HOW TO SUPPORT GOOD MELATONIN LEVELS

✓ Keep your bedroom as dark as possible.
✓ Reduce your exposure to bright artificial lights after sunset.
✓ Avoid LED lighting in the bedroom.
✓ The red-light spectrum is ideal for evening. This light mimics our natural human state of using firelight and candles while preparing for sleep and helps return our bodies to a restful state.

CHRONIC STRESS AND SLEEP

Poor-quality sleep can occur as a result of long-term stress. Conversely, it can also become a prime activator of the stress response. Sometimes the consequences of chronic sleep deprivation are seen within a few months of a disrupted sleep cycle.

CASE STUDY | KAREN

Sue

Sue had been seeing me for general women's business – such as pap smears and breast health checks – for about five years. Then, one visit she sat down in my office and uncharacteristically burst into tears.

She told me she couldn't sleep. I asked her to explain in more detail about the sleep issues she was having. It seemed that for around 20 years, from her late teens, she had been sleeping for a maximum of four to six hours per night. When she was younger, it did not appear to impact on her energy levels or her ability to complete her university degree. In fact, she hadn't really thought about her lack of sleep time as a problem until she read a recent article in a women's magazine about the consequences of insomnia on health.

I went through a checklist of known sleep saboteurs. She drank modestly but well within my optimal health limits for alcohol intake. Her bedroom was dark and quiet, and her husband slept like a baby without snoring. Her hormonal balance seemed fine, although her periods had become a little heavier when she hit 40 a year ago.

When I asked her how much coffee she drank, she replied: 'It can't be that. I've been drinking coffee since I started university.'

I explained the length of time caffeine can sit in the bloodstream. It can activate the adrenaline receptors on the brain for up to 18 hours. It will and can keep you bright and alert through the night like a meerkat on patrol. Sue's timeline of insomnia correlated with an increase in daily coffees – instead of one instant cup occasionally, she was now drinking two or three black espressos each morning.

Sue agreed to commit to stopping all caffeine for six weeks and to then come back for review. I warned her that she may get a caffeine withdrawal headache within the first few days and instructed her to load with magnesium phosphate tablets (65mg, four times daily) for the first four days to minimise the consequence of withdrawal and to help with sleep. I started her on melatonin to aid with good-quality sleep. I knew she was a little sceptical, but she was sufficiency concerned about her health to follow through with the plan.

On her return visit a few weeks later Sue was a different person. It took just five days for her to achieve seven hours of sleep, which was a record for her. She was looking and feeling more refreshed and had a smile on her face. Her blood pressure was a healthy 120/65 and pulse was down to 74.

YOUR CIRCADIAN RHYTHM

Put simply, your circadian rhythm is your natural sleep and wake cycle. It is affected by biochemical changes in your hormone profile. Human beings are daylight dwellers, and the circadian rhythm relies on this. We don't see well in the dark and we are not programmed to be a nocturnal species. Our ancestors had the moon, stars and fire at night for light. Without artificial light, humans generally rose early in the morning when the sun came up and prepared for sleep as the sun went down. Sleep probably happened well before midnight.

Your body is susceptible to light and dark. Daylight has a **blue spectrum** and evening light has a **red spectrum**. Your brain is sophisticated enough to use each spectrum, regardless of cloud cover. Each light spectrum initiates the production of biochemical messages that put you to sleep or wake you up.

The process that results in good sleep starts when the blue light of day activates your brain to send a signal to the gut. This signals the production of a neurological chemical that makes you feel good: serotonin.

It may surprise many to learn that more than 90 per cent of serotonin is made in your gut.

A healthy gut is essential for this process to happen and will provide the brain with optimum levels of serotonin required by your body each day.

As the light changes in the evening to a red-light spectrum, your brain then cleverly signals the conversion of serotonin to melatonin, the CEO of your sleep. It takes approximately four hours for this conversion to happen. Ideally, you should be in bed asleep or going to sleep within four hours of sunset. To support this, the hours before bed should be lit by soft, dimmed lights and candles. Fire is the exact red light that assists our body's conversion from awake to asleep.

Artificial light interferes with this natural process, including the light on technological devices, because it has a blue-light spectrum. Light toxicity is the term used when artificial light interferes with the natural biochemical rhythms required for sleep. If you are not sleeping, you will need to rehabilitate this vital process which will mean sacrificing some of your usual habits. A good night's sleep every night is worth the effort for your health, happiness and productivity at home and in the workplace.

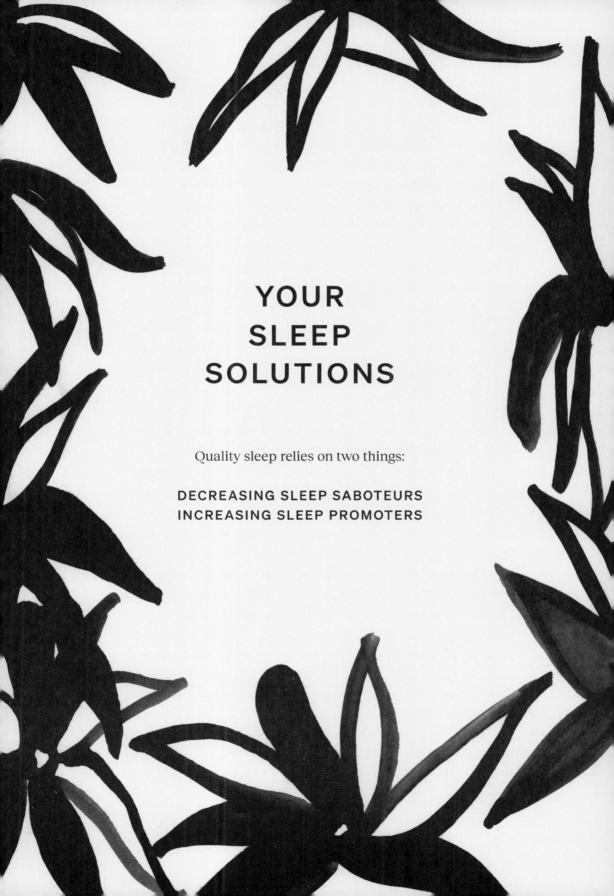

YOUR
SLEEP
SOLUTIONS

Quality sleep relies on two things:

DECREASING SLEEP SABOTEURS
INCREASING SLEEP PROMOTERS

Sleep saboteurs

If you are not sleeping,
employ the following recommendations.

REMOVE STIMULANTS

Cut out caffeine completely for a while. Caffeine is found in coffee, carbonated drinks and chocolate. You can reintroduce them to your routine when you start sleeping well again, but cap coffee at two cups per day and drink them before noon. Limit chocolate to 20g after midday unless you sleep like a baby.

Cut out alcohol completely for a while. Alcohol makes you drowsy and helps you fall asleep. However, when your liver starts its cycle of natural detoxification during sleep, you may wake up and be unable to sleep for a few hours. Alcohol can also interrupt sleep for men over the age of 35 years and menopausal women, due to its irritant effect on the bladder.

Cacao and cocoa are stimulants and contain 240mg caffeine per 100g (the equivalent of three espresso coffees!) so please remove these from your diet during your rehab phase.

AVOID SUGAR

A diet high in sugar - whether it's in your food or what you drink - will impact sleep quality. It's a vicious cycle - poor sleep means you have reduced energy levels, so you may reach for sugary foods and drinks for 'false energy' to get you through the day. Which then means... you guessed it, a poor night's sleep. Try to avoid sugary foods at least four hours before bedtime with the ultimate goal to reduce your sugar intake overall.

REDUCE MENTAL AND EMOTIONAL STIMULATION

Decreasing stress will help promote good-quality sleep. Levels of the stress hormone cortisol should be naturally low during sleep. Cortisol surges around sunrise, switching off the melatonin and allowing you to gently wake up. If this hormone is elevated due to mental and emotional pressure, it may reach its peak in the early hours and switch off melatonin before sunrise, leaving you wide awake before the birds are up. See Chapters 7 and 8 for advice on reducing your stress hormones.

Avoid confrontations or any mental agitation before bed. Arguing with family members, reading work emails or worrying about deadlines may produce adrenaline. This means that the body will keep sleep at bay if danger is present, whether this danger is real or perceived.

Try to introduce some positive habits – meditation, breathing exercises and warm baths can calm your mind and help your body understand it is safe to sleep.

REDUCE LIGHT TOXICITY

✓ Use dimmers on your lights at night and include candlelight (preferably beeswax candles) if possible.

✓ Avoid using backlit devices and watching screens such as the TV, mobile or tablets and bright lights two hours before bed.

✓ Use blackout curtains and blinds to block all light from artificial sources outside your home.

✓ Remove all light from your bedroom. Even the light of a device on standby or a softly lighted clock may interfere with your natural internal rhythm.

✓ Try to rise with the light of the day. Wherever possible, be outside at sunrise or just after this time. This will stimulate your system to sync with its natural rhythm in sequence with the sun. After a while you will naturally wake up and be able to avoid using alarms. The word itself is jarring, it literally 'alarms' you from your sleep!

Sleep promoters

The following suggestions work best in conjunction with removing the saboteurs that may be affecting your sleep.

✓ Create a regular routine. When you're busy, it can feel like there are not enough hours in the day, that using the hours after dinner is your only option. If you are not sleeping well, this habit needs to change.

✓ Have dinner by 7pm to allow time for digestion.

✓ Create a ritual before bed: wash, stretch, meditate, use soft lighting, aromatherapy oils, warm herbal tea, or make love. These are all good ways to relax.

✓ Be in bed asleep or going to sleep no later than 11pm. Early birds will need to ensure that their bedtime allows for an eight-hour sleep.

✓ Count backwards from when you need to wake up and ensure you're in bed with enough time to allow seven to eight hours of sleep. This is crucial and takes discipline. Make the commitment to yourself.

✓ Leave your phone on flight mode at night to prevent being disturbed (better still, leave it outside the bedroom while you are sleeping).

✓ If you wake through the night, avoid switching on any bright lights. Invest in a very soft night-light or use a candle. Make a cup of caffeine-free herbal tea - this will have a calming effect on the nervous system. Try passionflower, Tulsa or chamomile. Drink it in bed, then roll over and breathe deeply, concentrating on your breathing. This will calm your nervous system and hopefully ease you back to sleep.

CLEAN UP YOUR SLEEP HYGIENE

It is estimated that humans sleep for approximately 203, 804 hours over a 70-year life span. In other words, one-third of our life is designed to be spent sleeping. It stands to reason that our sleep environment is an essential element to enhance our ability to have quality sleep.

Ready to take charge of your sleep? Here's where to start to improve your State of Being (whatever stage you're in).

✓ Your bedroom needs to be used just for sleeping and making love.

✓ Remove all electronic devices, including television sets and digital devices.

✓ Turn off your Wi-Fi at night.

✓ Natural ventilation is preferable. Use a fan, open your bedroom windows, or have a cool shower before bed, rather than turning on the air conditioning.

✓ Vacuum the floor and dust the surfaces regularly to avoid inhaling irritants while you sleep.

✓ Invest in a good mattress; they last about 10 years.

✓ Invest in a good pillow that suits your frame; they last about five years.

✓ Use cotton or natural fibre bed linen. Blankets and duvets should be made from natural fibres such as wool, bamboo, silk, hemp and cotton.

✓ Your body temperature is essential to quality sleep – if it's too hot or too cold, you will wake up. Sleep studies suggest a slightly cooler environment is more conducive to a good night's sleep.

MEDICAL REASONS YOUR SLEEP MAY BE POOR

SLEEP APNOEA

Poor sleep is sometimes due to an obstruction in the airway. Someone who snores, for example, will be experiencing some form of disruption from mild to extreme. This should be investigated by a sleep study. Sleep GPs are Medical GPs with a special interest in sleep and provide an integrated approach, often offering a sleep study you can experience in your own home.

Snoring partners can be one of the biggest saboteurs to good-quality sleep. Encourage them to address their sleep quality and make sleep quality a partnership project as you will both benefit from this.

Once you re-establish your quality sleep, slowly introduce your previous habits, one by one, and pay attention to any that irritate your quality sleep pattern. It is then your choice as to how you proceed. Our advice is to remove these irritants permanently, or at least significantly reduce them.

HORMONAL BALANCE

This is essential for quality sleep. PMS and menopause can interfere with our sleep cycle, particularly if the hormone progesterone is compromised in some way as this hormone promotes sleep. Working with an integrated GP and specialised naturopath can help you regain hormonal balance with lifestyle adjustments, supplements and, if needed, natural hormone replacements.

MENOPAUSE AND SLEEP

When I began to enter menopause, I noticed a change in my sleep habits common with this hormonal transition. I found acupuncture from Chinese Medicine and natural progesterone cream from my integrated GP (Dr Karen, of course!) were both essential support for my sleep. Today, I sleep really well with no medication, apart from some melatonin that I keep on hand for travel. (In Australia, melatonin is available through pharmacies on prescription from a doctor or over the counter if you are over 55).

I will have a wakeful night occasionally, but there's always a reason why: an extra glass of wine with friends, too late to bed, dessert, or sometimes the full moon or a loud storm. Disturbed sleep after a celebration is not a problem on the odd occasion, but will sabotage your ability to maintain a thriving state if it becomes a regular habit.

I have learnt that as long as I support my own natural rhythms and avoid overdoing what I know interferes with my sleep, I have good-quality sleep worth cheering about.

PARTNERS

Partners who snore or fidget in their sleep can disturb you. If you are a good sleeper and your partner is disturbing your sleep, putting them into sleep rehabilitation is the best option for all concerned. Sleep apnoea or other irritants may be preventing them from sleeping deeply and this will be affecting their health, moods and performance in life.

BABIES AND CHILDREN

If the reason your sleep is interrupted is unavoidable, such as attending to a baby, try to nap during the day when they do (as much as possible) rather than cooking and cleaning as soon as they are asleep. Your emotional ability to be present with your child depends on you getting enough sleep. It is worth noting that breastfeeding will provide mothers with an ideal level of progesterone and this has a protective mechanism to negate many of the harmful effects of insomnia.

PETS

If a pet is preventing you from sleeping, or from sleeping well, you need to remove them from the bedroom. We know this can be very challenging, however your sleep is essential. If you love your cats, remember they tend to sleep all day and like to play at night. Dogs of course just take over the bed and push you into a tiny area. Be honest, would you sleep better if your pets did not sleep with you? It may take a while and some convincing before they accept the new rules. Try to create a morning routine of love and attention instead.

SHIFT WORKERS AND SLEEP

Let's start with a heartfelt thank you, as shift workers are usually involved in emergency services, health care or another service that supports humans. Sadly, however, this is a huge disruption to your natural rhythm and you may already experience some of the side effects such as increased fat gain. Unfortunately, it does not stop there. Shift work can increase your financial gain, but in the long term, you can pay a big price on your health. Research shows shift workers have an increased risk of all-cause mortality. Ideally, as you get older, depending on your genetic predisposition and your health challenges, it may pay in the long run to rethink this aspect of your working life in a way that could benefit your health.

There are things you can do to reduce the impact as much as possible if you are doing shift work. All other areas of your lifestyle need to be as ideal as possible: nutrition, movement, activation of the Blue Zone (re-read Chapters 6, 7 and 8 if necessary) and reduce toxicity (alcohol and caffeine) to support your body to deal with the high demand of being out of sync with its natural design. If you have a leaky gut or food intolerances and other digestive disorders, it is worthwhile working with a naturopath to improve your gut health.

SHIFT WORK SLEEP SOLUTIONS

- Make sure you have time in darkened rooms before attempting to sleep.

- Wear earplugs, so you're less likely to be disturbed.

- Afternoon naps before work are beneficial.

- Try to work in a regular rhythm – keep your rooms as dark as possible during the day with dimmed artificial light or candlelight to simulate night.

- Invest in blackout curtains or blinds to keep daylight completely out of the room where you sleep during the day.

- Walk, move or exercise before you go to work. Consider a yin-style movement option when you have finished work to assist your nervous system to settle before you go to sleep (such as yoga, tai chi, Qi Gong, light Pilates).

- Talk to your GP about a prescription for melatonin to ensure you have the CEO on board before you settle for your night (in the day).

- Get seven to eight hours quality sleep every 24 hours.

- Drink plenty of water, but reduce the amount you drink four hours before you go to sleep. This will reduce your bladder activity during sleep.

SEASONAL SLEEP

You may notice that your sleep patterns shift with the seasons. It's natural to want to sleep more in winter as the nights get darker early and the sun rises later in the morning. In summer, if you are in a good circadian rhythm, you may naturally wake around 5am. In winter, you may not wake until an hour or so later. If your lifestyle can support this need to sleep longer, it is ideal to follow this natural tendency in the colder winter months.

INTERNATIONAL TRAVEL AND JETLAG

Make the most of your overseas travel. Look for clever apps that advise you how to minimise jet lag on arrival at your new time zone. Good sleep preparation starts a few days before boarding a plane. The technology in apps like Timeshifter (**timeshifter.com**) uses research from NASA that promotes good sleep cycles in astronauts. In the future, we may see this research adopted by progressive airlines in changes to inflight cabin light, food and sleep schedules to prepare passengers biorhythms so they arrive refreshed and more aligned with their destination time zone.

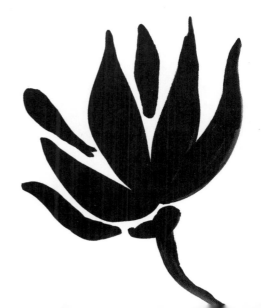

SLEEP SUPPORT AND YOUR DIET

What you eat can have a huge bearing on your sleep cycle and the quality of your sleep. The following foods contain the protein building blocks needed to build good levels of our sleep hormone melatonin, along with the co-factor foods that convert food protein into melatonin.

Pistachio nuts have been shown to contain trace amounts of melatonin. Around 30g, or a small palmful, of these nuts provide a nutritious evening snack that may also enhance quality sleep.

Choose a variety of these types of foods every day and chew them well before swallowing. If you don't get this foundation right, chances are you will end up spending time dozing in a doctor's waiting room.

PROTEIN CHOICES	CO-FACTOR FOODS
Fish	Oysters
Chicken	Cocoa
Turkey	Brazil nuts
Eggs	Berries
Dairy	Tomatoes
Pepitas	Buckwheat
Walnuts	Spinach
Soy	Parsley

HERBAL HELP

The herbs hops and valerian are good places to start when it comes to supporting a good night of sleep. German research combines these two to help initiate sleep and then keep you there until you find Deep Sleep.

Other herbs that can help are **Zizyphus** and **Withania Somnifera**. These can often be found in combination herbal products from naturopathic health food stores.

Melatonin can also be a great insomnia buster. This can be sourced online or from a local doctor on prescription (or can be obtained over the counter in a pharmacy if you are aged over 55). The adult dose is 2 to 6mg taken one to two hours before bed. Some doctors will also prescribe this in liquid form – the suggested dose is 10mg per ml. The nightly dose for drops is 10 to 15 drops at bedtime.

GABA can also help for sleep disturbed by anxiety. The dose is 200mg at bedtime and a second dose of 100mg if you wake after midnight.

If sleep problems persist, visit a naturopath, Chinese Medical practitioner, integrated doctor or Sleep GP. Sometimes, if insomnia is severe and prolonged, your doctor may consider a short course of sleeping tablets. It's still important to work on your sleep solutions even if medication is needed for a little while.

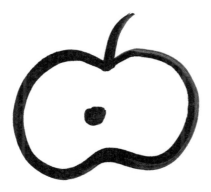

What's next?

Moving forward with Pillar Five

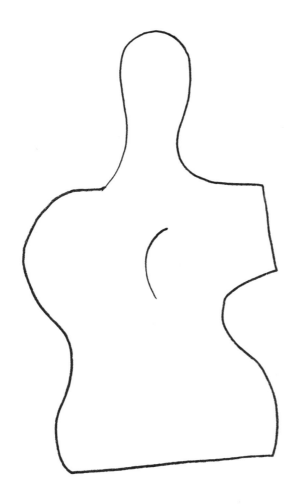

10.
THRIVING IN
A TOXIC WORLD

I like
my products like
I like my people.
Non-toxic.

FOLLAIN

Are you curious to know whether the choices you make in your daily life increase your risk of cancer and diseases such as cardiovascular disease, dementia, Parkinson's, autoimmune disease and fertility problems?

The following questions focus on the potential exposure you have with the multiple chemicals and ionising radiation existing in your life.

The traditional belief that 'the dose maketh the poison' does not apply when we start to understand and focus on the impact of chemicals on cellular pathways of health. Genetic studies on the efficiency of gene pathways within every cell of our body are now showing damage from chemicals like Bisphenol A at levels far below what was previously considered the 'safe' human exposure level.

Genes you inherited from your parents are interacting with the chemicals from our environment for the first time in human history.

80 per cent of your total body load of chemicals comes through your food source, *and it's been this way since the 1940s.*

But how safe are these chemicals that are only valuable to high-intensity farming?

Safe pesticide levels are determined by health regulators using animal studies based on presumptions dating from the 1950s. All studies use extrapolated data assumptions based on studies in rats. In order to determine safe human levels of a chemical known to cause death at certain levels, rats are fed increasing concentrations of the chemical until 50 per cent of them die. This level of chemical is labelled the LD50 of that particular toxin: i.e. the lethal dose that killed 50 per cent of the subjects. From here, a mathematical calculation is taken, resulting in the determination of 'safe' levels in humans for use in food, on food and in the air.

Ask yourself the question, 'Does a little bit of poison matter, when it comes to the food I eat?' The answer actually depends on how robust your genes work. The emerging science of **Nutrigenomics** (see Chapter 11) looks at how a person's gene expression interacts with the food they eat (and chemicals they ingest) and points to a huge fault in the logic of this process to determine the safety of chemicals. For example, we know that some women who have inherited less efficient detox pathways carry a much greater health burden when chemicals are mixed with hormones.

Inflammation is the driver of all chronic disease. As you age, the efficiency of your genetic detox pathways slows down and makes it even more important to reduce your toxic load. As more of these man-made chemicals accumulate, these demon molecules will then hunt down variations in genes and turn up inflammation to screaming levels. In women, many of these chemicals like BPA and phthalates are hormone disruptors that start a domino of unhealthy changes in our fertility hormone dance and increases the risk of cancer. In athletes, this also impacts on recovery time from exercise and increases the risk of injury from heavy training sessions.

TOXIC LOAD AUDIT

This audit is best used as a baseline to judge your improved lifestyle options and reduced chemical burden as you embark your journey toward a **Thriving State of Being**.

There is only the option of Yes or No answers. There is no option for sometimes or maybe. It is intended to focus on the impact of things we do regularly that are 'normal' in our community, that increases your toxic chemical body burden. Any YES answers will impact health – for those who are genetically resilient this impact will be lower than for those who have inherited less efficient pathways of chemical removal.

	YES	NO
Do you smoke?		
Do you allow smoking in your home?		
On average do you watch television more than 10 hours per week?		
On average do use a computer more than 10 hours per week?		
Do you have foam cushions in your bedroom or living areas?		
Do you use a pod coffeemaker?		
Is your mattress treated with a soil or stain-protectant?		
Do you use perfumed air fresheners at home?		
Do you have a deodoriser in your car?		
Do you have pressed-wood furniture (usually assemble-yourself items) in your home or office?		

	YES	NO
Do you wrap leftovers and other food items with plastic wrap?		
Do you cook with non-stick pots or frying pans, other than Eco-pans?		
Do you re-use plastic water bottles?		
Do you eat tinned food? Canned tuna? Add an extra ONE point.		
Do you microwave food or drinks in plastic containers or with a plastic-wrap covering?		
Do you drink town water (chlorinated water) straight from the tap?		
Do you use hairspray, mousse or hair gel?		
Do you use perfume or cologne?		
Do you use spray deodorant?		
Do your moisturisers, body lotions or sunscreen contain Parabens?		
Do you use dry-cleaning services more than two or three times per year?		
Do you have weekly contact with plastic or vinyl toys?		
Do you use antibacterial kitchen bench sprays?		
Do you have ant or cockroach baits in the house?		
Are insect sprays used in your home?		
Do you work with farm or garden sprays, chemicals or pesticides?		
Do you handle EFTPOS receipts?		
Do you spend more than four days per week indoors?		
Do you live on a main road?		
Do you live under the flight path of an airport?		
Do you often drive a car or take public transport in heavy traffic?		
Have you purchased a brand-new car within the last 12 months?		
Does your home have wall-to-wall synthetic carpeting?		
Do you have vinyl flooring in the kitchen or bathroom?		
Do any rooms in your house have wallpaper?		
Do you fly in an airplane more than twice per year?		
Do you use your mobile phone for more than one hour per day?		
Do you sit at a computer monitor for more than one hour per day?		
Has your home had a termite or pest treatment in the last five years?		
Have your carpets been professionally cleaned in the last 12 months?		

	YES	NO
Do you use dry-cleaning agents in your job?		
Do you work in the nail or hairdressing industry?		
Do you work as a motor mechanic?		
Have you ever worked with mercury (for example, in dentistry)?		

HOW TO CALCULATE YOUR SCORE

Score **ONE** point for every **YES** answer.
Subtract **FIVE** points if approximately half the food you eat is organically farmed.
Subtract **TEN** points if more than **80** per cent of your food is organically sourced.
Subtract **FIVE** points if your personal care items (shampoo, conditioner and skincare) are organically certified.

YOUR FINAL SCORE _____

0 – 5 POINTS

You have a clean lifestyle and a low risk for environmental health challenges. Congratulations for making great choices for you and your family. Keep up the good work!

6 – 10 POINTS

You are doing better than average, but some improvements may make a difference to your health in the future. Continue reading this chapter for some suggestions on where you can make some changes.

10 – 20 POINTS

Making some effort and changes now may mean that you dodge a disease-bullet. This chapter outlines some easy-to-follow suggestions and solutions to help you implement some changes.

20-PLUS POINTS

Eek! Consider this your wake-up call. It's time to do some work to reduce your chances of spending a lot of time in doctor's waiting rooms in the future. There is no better time to start than right NOW!

Review the questions where you answered 'Yes' on the audit. Take special note of **Questions One** through **28**. These areas of exposure are, for the most part, under your direct control. By following the guidelines below, you will reduce your score and your toxic burden within **two weeks.**

This will give you some breathing space to deal with the chemicals associated with the remaining audit questions (**questions 29 through 45**). These areas require more effort to affect change.

TOXIC LOAD SOLUTIONS

Regardless of your toxic load score and/or your State of Being, there are some simple changes you can make to ensure that your environment, your home, your diet and your lifestyle choices are as healthy and toxin-free as possible.

FOOD, FOOD STORAGE AND REDUCING THE TOXIC LOAD

The move to organically harvested foods can eliminate more than 80 per cent of the chemicals entering your body. Review **Chapter 3** to remind yourself about the importance of making organic food choices. At a minimum, foods such as berries and leafy greens need to be organically sourced.

1   **Source organic produce**. A huge number of studies show this alone can reduce the body chemical load by over 80 per cent. Try farmers' markets, organic sections of your supermarket, health food stores, independent grocers or try to grow some of your own organic ingredients to enjoy.

2   **Avoid food wrap and plastic containers**. Most are impregnated with members of the Bisphenol family, proven to disrupt the finely tuned dance of fertility hormones. Heating food in plastic causes chemicals to leach into the heated food at a much faster rate. Move to glass storage containers and invest in beeswax food covers. Beeswax covers can be rinsed and reused so are an ideal alternative to standard food wraps.

3   **Invest in a drip coffee maker**. The current fad of pod coffeemakers exposes the drinker to the heated aluminium that is pierced to allow the pod to release its coffee. Switch to a more traditional method of coffee making. Drip filter coffee has been proven to provide the most antioxidant supply of all methods of coffee making, without the nasties.

REDUCE YOUR HOME'S TOXIC LOAD

1   **Replace soft furnishings as they age**. Choose natural fillers like cotton, featherdown or wool fibres. If you use any other type of pillow for sleeping, triple bag it with extra pillow slips.

2   **Declutter the compounds**. There are more than 4000 different synthetic organofluorine compounds, a chemical group known as PFAS (per- and polyfluoroalkyl substances). These compounds persist unaltered and indefinitely in both nature and the human body. They have been around since the 1940s and can accumulate in human tissue over time. Despite a push to phase these guys out of production in 2018, they can still be found in the following everyday household items:

- ✗ scotch-guarded fabrics for waterproofing
- ✗ spill-proofing sprays for soft furnishings
- ✗ cookware
- ✗ plastic food containers
- ✗ mattresses (use a natural fibre protector that can be regularly cleaned and doesn't carry the risk of chemical residue)

3   **Clear the air naturally**. Air fresheners, deodorisers, perfumes and other spray personal items are one of the highest sources of environmental pollution, exceeding car emissions. The interior of a home carries a higher burden of volatile organic compounds than outdoors. Eliminate the use of any product that comes in a pressurised spray pack. Source natural essential oils for perfume alternatives. Use natural citrus-based liquids for a fresher smell in the kitchen and living areas.

4   **Clean naturally**. Use a natural cleanser based on vinegar and bicarbonate of soda instead of chemical sprays. Making your own cleaning solutions will not only save money, but you'll also protect your family's health. Use the money you've saved by making your own cleaning products and spend this money on buying organic food instead.

5   **Become a plant person**. Reduce the amount of airborne chemicals with indoor plants. Weeping fig and Fatsia Japonica remove 80 per cent of formaldehyde in as little as four hours after being introduced to a room. Mother-in-Law Tongue is also worthy of honourable mention. It is a hardy plant that can go for up to four weeks without watering and still perform its air-cleaning role.

6   **Consider natural woods**. Encourage the use of natural woods for furniture rather than compressed melamine products. The adhesive used in most prefabricated pressed-wood products emit volatile chemicals for more than 12 months.

7   **Treat your body well**. Read the labels on all personal care items – what goes **on** the skin, goes **in**. Avoid products which list chemicals, preservatives and ingredients not sourced from nature. Avoid products that list parabens as an ingredient. There are other chemicals that create a free radical load on the skin cells, creating accelerated ageing over time, but the paraben family is particularly toxic. A good resource when shopping for personal care and beauty items is Safe Cosmetics Australia (**safecosmeticsaustralia.com.au**).

IMPORTANT!
Reduce all exposure to cigarette smoke. If you were a
smoker before picking up this book, commit to give up today.
Congratulate yourself on taking the amazing step towards
a **Thriving State of Being**.

COMPUTERS AND YOUR TOXIC LOAD

1   **Reduce the amount of time spent in front of the television**. These
machines emit electromagnetic radiation along with blue light. These
lights may impact your ability to achieve a deep restorative sleep. Sit as
far away from the TV as possible and avoid the temptation of installing
one in the bedroom.

2   **Cut down on computer use**. The same rules for televisions apply to
computer use. These are best used early in the day and put to bed at
sundown. Beware of laptop use, particularly in bed or sitting on the sofa.
This exposes the delicate ovaries to an extra dose of electromagnetic
radiation. Although there is no evidence at present that this poses
a problem, common sense would suggest that this is not a good thing.

3   **Turn off your Wi-Fi at the source in the evening**. This can have
positive flow-on effects for children, who may then turn to a book for
company rather than the latest downloadable game craze. Children
are particularly vulnerable to the negative effects of blue light on their
sleep patterns.

4   **Activate the night mode on smartphones from 8pm**. Most modern
smartphones have this option. The screen will switch to a more sleep-
friendly shade of red hues, rather than a stimulating blue screen.

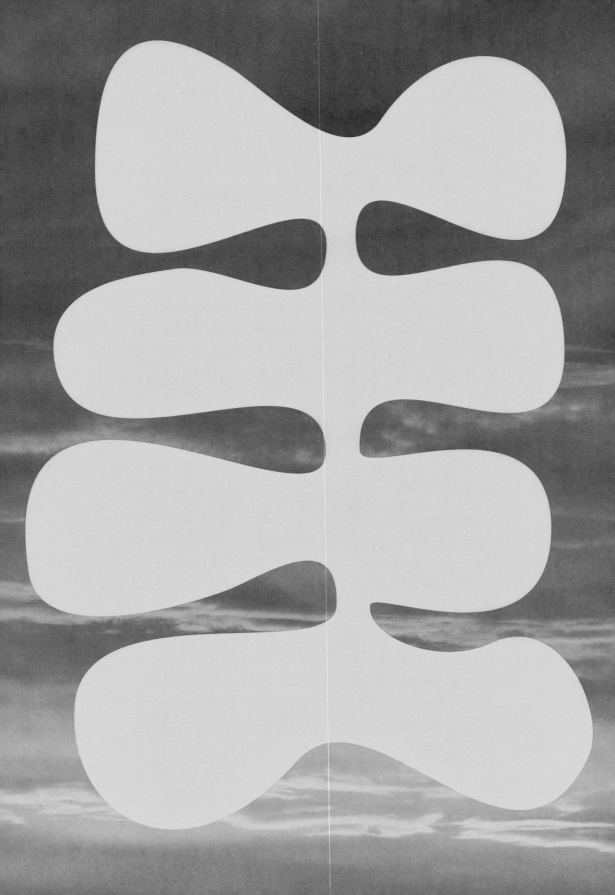

DECIPHERING RECYCLING NUMBERS

Numbers appearing in triangles on plastic items are not strictly speaking recycling numbers. They are used to indicate the type of plastic used to make the item. This information then indicates whether that product can be repurposed by the recycling industry. More importantly, it gives consumers clues on how to use these chemically based products safely.

PETE OR POLYETHYLENE TEREPHTHALATE

Found in:
- plastic soft drink bottles
- bottled water in plastic containers
- fruit juice containers
- plastic cooking oil containers
- some medications
- medical equipment

Phthalates are unstable in plastic and easily transfer to air, or to the food or cosmetic in contact with it. If present in skincare items, it can be absorbed directly into the bloodstream.

Studies show some children contain 20 times the recommended 'safe' level of this chemical in their blood, but no lower limit of safety has been firmly established.

Phthalates been found in the urine of pregnant women and linked to increased blood pressure and alterations in the health of blood vessel walls in both adults and children. Those carrying gene variants in cardiovascular gene pathways will be more vulnerable to this chemical.

Strategies to minimise exposure:
- Avoid all food in contact with this chemical
- Buy food and drinks in glass containers

HDPE OR HIGH-DENSITY POLYETHYLENE

HDPE is cost-effective and easily recyclable, making it an attractive option for the container manufacturing industry. This plastic makes more sturdy containers for supermarket items like milk and cooking oil, dishwashing and laundry detergents. You may also find it in the haircare section containing shampoos and body soaps. Because of its hardwearing properties it is also a favourite for outdoor furniture, rubbish bins and raised garden beds.

Strategies to minimise exposure:
- Recycle products labelled with this chemical to reduce its environmental impact
- Avoid all personal care or food items packaged with this label

PVC OR POLYVINYL CHLORIDE

This chemical makes plastic soft and flexible. Most households will have an extensive list of products containing PVC. It is found in most kitchens as food or plastic wrap for leftovers. It is also used extensively in the food industry as trays for supermarket-packaged fruit and vegetables. It is used in pet and children's toys and teething rings.

Most modern homes will used PVC pipes to deliver water to the household. Garden hoses maintain their flexibility with PVC. These products continue to leach chemicals as they age. They are not recyclable, so are a huge burden on the environment.

Strategies to minimise exposure:
- Never buy or use PVC goods in contact with food, pets or children
- Source children's toys made from soft, natural fibres
- Buy reusable beeswax covers for food and leftovers
- Invest in a water filter for all household use
- Source a PVC-free garden hose made of the more stable Polyurethane

LDPE OR LOW-DENSITY POLYETHYLENE

Australia is already leading the way in reducing the impact of this chemical, found in supermarket plastic bags, shrink wrap for food and soft plastic sandwich bags. You will find it in the soft plastic bags used to wrap sliced bread in bakeries and in the produce bags offered for loose fruit and vegetables in the supermarket It is also used in containers for squeeze bottle condiments like tomato sauce.

Strategies to reduce health and environmental impact:
- Carry reusable cloth bags for grocery and food shopping
- Buy condiments packaged in glass containers
- Use (and reuse) paper bags for fruit and vegetable shopping
- Reuse plastic bags at home
- Use baking paper and paper bags to wrap children's lunch items

PP OR POLYPROPYLENE

This creates a more rigid packaging product (think of the internal package of a processed cereal) that keeps the product airtight within the cardboard container. It is also found in plastic bottle tops and food containers for margarines and yoghurts. They are also found in disposable nappies.

These are recyclable and relatively heat stable, but only 3 per cent of polypropylene products make it to the recycling centre.

Strategies to minimise exposure:
- Avoid highly processed food
- Make your own cereals from organically sourced products and store in glass containers.
- Recycle containers
- Use cloth nappies

POLYSTYRENE

Items made from polystyrene, like disposable foam cups, drinking straws and cutlery, are gradually being phased out of use in Australia because of environmental concerns. When heated, styrene, a carcinogen, can leach into food from containers. This is not a recyclable product and should be avoided.

INCLUDES BPA PLASTICS AND OTHER 'LEFTOVER' CHEMICALS.

Most plastics in this category are not recyclable. The most potent is the Bisphenol family. Bisphenols have been extensively researched and are known endocrine disruptors that can mimic our own hormones (they are xeno-oestrogens) and create havoc with our health and fertility. Until recently they were the main plastic used in drink bottles and baby formula bottles. BPA is now still found in thermal paper for EFTPOS receipts.

Strategies to minimise exposure:
- Never drink or eat from plastic containers labelled BPA
- Avoid handling EFTPOS receipts or wash hands thoroughly before eating if you have to handle these types of receipts often

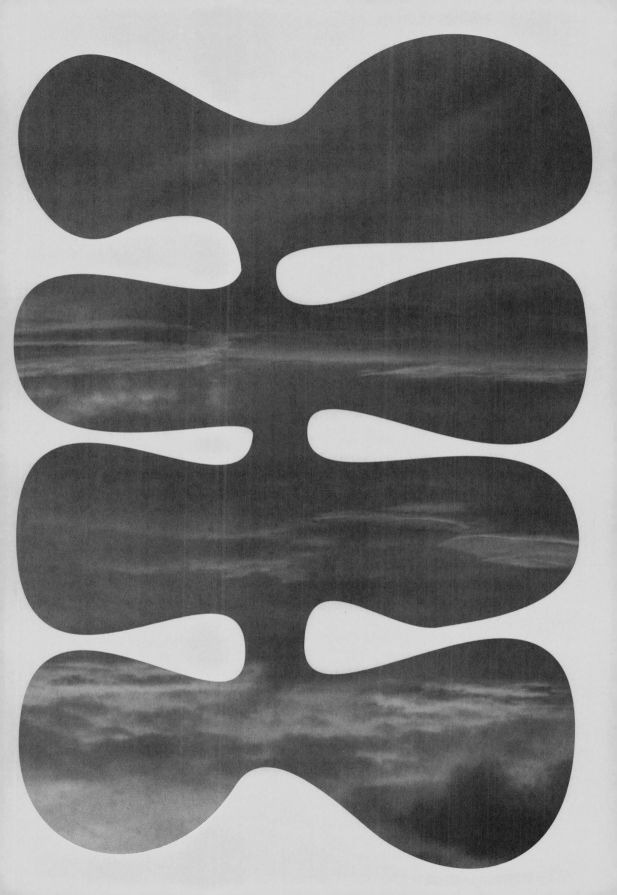

A WORD ABOUT MICRO-PLASTICS

You should always rinse rice well before cooking. This nutritious and natural food may be contaminated with up to 35mg of tiny micro-plastic particles per 100 grams. These micro-plastics will rapidly break down during the cooking process to release multiple chemicals that will impact human health. Avoid 'instant rice' as this form of rice contains an even greater micro-plastic load and has already been subjected to high heat in the preparation process.

BISPHENOL GROUP OF CHEMICALS – A DISHONOURABLE MENTION

Karen says: 'In May 2012, I read an article on the website of Food Standards Australia New Zealand (FSANZ) about the safety of a group of chemicals known as Bisphenols (BPAs), which are mixed with plastics to increase the flexibility of the product. The FSANZ is a government-funded organisation responsible for determining safe levels of chemicals in food fit for human consumption in Australia. Entitled "The Dose Maketh the Poison", the paper was an essay on the safety of all approved chemicals in the food industry based on this premise, despite there being an increasing number of studies in the genetic field suggesting the opposite. As a nutritionally trained medical doctor, the article alarmed me on several fronts. I wrote to the author of the paper, the Chief Scientist of Food Standards Australia, with a list of current research papers that countered the arguments for safety contained in the article. Not surprisingly I received no reply. When I checked in 2016, the article had been removed from the website and BPA has now been recognised by Government as a significant hormone disruptor and threat to human health at very low levels. I see this time and time again, where robust research precedes changes in policy in most cases by decades.'

BPA and other chemicals disrupt the natural biochemical flow and balance of hormonal pathways in the human body. These chemicals are enemies of optimal wellness.

REDUCE BPA BURDEN

These solutions could reduce BPA body burden by over 60 per cent in just seven days.

1   Use paper or glass containers instead of plastic wrap for food storage. Baking paper and beeswax wraps are a great alternative to plastic wrap. You can also wrap food in baking paper before placing in plastic containers.

2   Do not re-use plastic water bottles.

3   Make sure that any food in contact with plastic is not heated. This includes microwaving. Instead, use a microwaveable or glass container.

4   Be careful with any plastic container labelled #7 for recycling as BPA plastics all carry this number (but not all plastics labelled #7 is BPA).

5   Be aware that tinned foods may be sealed with BPAs. Tinned tuna, tinned salmon and tinned fruit are the most commonly affected, so minimise or eliminate these (or look for tins that state they are BPA free).

6   Avoid handling thermal paper, including EFTPOS receipts. as these are impregnated with BPAs. If your work involves handling these items, wash your hands regularly.

7   Consider installing a home water-filtration system for your drinking water. A carbon block and titanium system will remove heavy metals, bacteria and parasites such as chlorine, BPA, benzenes and trihalomethanes. You can find options for less than $150.

8   Maintain pristine condition of your liver to aid the elimination of BPA and other toxins. Revisit Chapter 4 for liver support strategies.

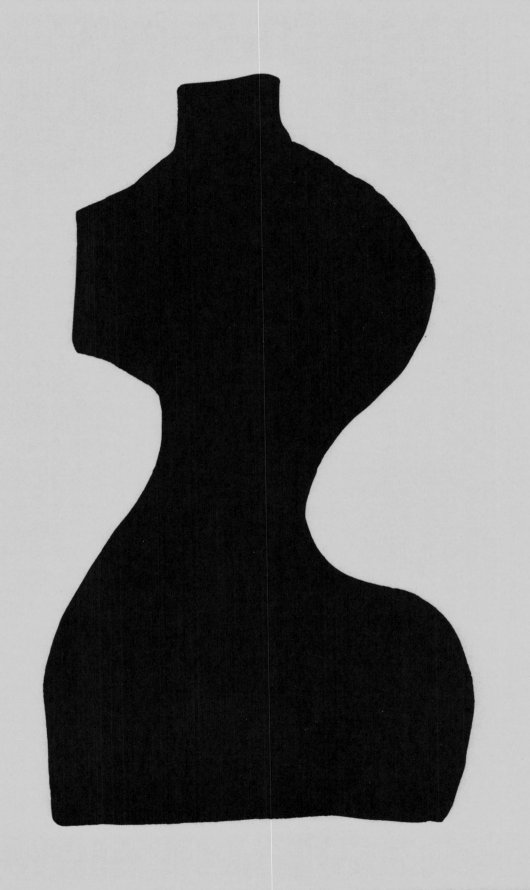

11.
SECRET WOMEN'S BUSINESS - FINDING HORMONAL HARMONY

Your period is not your enemy. On the contrary, it's a sound barometer of your overall health.

KIRSTEN KARCHMER

Why is it that a normally placid woman can become so exhausted and irritable prior to her menstrual cycle that she transforms into a suffering and vicious she-wolf? Why can she begin snapping and snarling at anyone unlucky enough to be in her path?

HORMONES: A FAMILIAR STORY

Karen says, 'During my early career in women's health I saw dozens of young women each month who would describe how their menstrual bleeding was preceded by varying lengths of irritability and mood swings, accompanied by sore breasts that doctors cleverly label "mastalgia".

'This trifecta of symptoms was literally the only one I encountered both personally as a busy and stressed newly graduated doctor, and as a common pattern in my female patients. I was so familiar with the story that one-by-one, I would reassure these women that their premenstrual symptoms of irritability, fatigue and breast tenderness were "normal". I would warn partners of these women to hide the kitchen knives at "that time of the month", and not take it personally. Sometimes, with no other choice in my clinical toolbox, I would offer the oral contraceptive pill as a solution for these women.

'It was only after I discovered the explanation for these symptoms, and the disruption of the intricate balance of the fertility hormone dance that I became armed with knowledge. The knowledge to help these young women out of their monthly hormonal nightmare without reaching for the prescription pad.'

THE FACTS

On any given day 800 million women in the world have their period.

60 per cent of women experience emotional and physical symptoms at some stage in their life before menstruating.

Five to 10 per cent of women suffer from PMDD.

HOW HORMONES WORK (AND DON'T!)

The medical profession is only just beginning to scratch the surface when it comes to unravelling the causes of hormonal havoc. There is good evidence however, that the 'Jekyll and Hyde' transformation which afflicts over 60 per cent of females in the Western world is related to a dominance of the female hormone known as oestrogen along with a deficiency in the amount of the more user-friendly female hormone called progesterone.

In order to unravel the mystery of female hormone balance, we need to look at what is 'normal', but may not, necessarily, be 'natural'.

OESTROGEN AND PROGESTERONE

One of the most important aspects is the ebb and flow of two fertility cycle hormones: oestrogen and progesterone. The absolute levels of these fertility hormones vary over a woman's phase, but perform a delicate balancing act with each other during a natural menstrual cycle.

Even in a post-menopausal life, there is an intrinsic balance between oestrogen and progesterone. Although they will then be at a consistently low baseline, these two hormones are still measurable on blood tests in older women and should have a healthy relationship to each other.

Let's explore the role of the two main fertility hormones in a woman.

THE ROLE OF OESTROGEN

- Retains body fluid
- Thickens the lining of the uterus in preparation for a pregnancy
- Plays a role in brain cognitive function, especially learning and memory
- Enhances communication skills
- Regulates appetite
- Enhances quality sleep
- Supports good bone density

THE ROLE OF PROGESTERONE

- Modulates the effect of oestrogen in the luteal phase (second half) of the menstrual cycle
- Hormonal support for a pregnancy in the first 12 to 14 weeks
- Thyroid support hormone
- Supports healthy breast tissue
- Mood stabiliser
- Natural antidepressant
- Releases body fluid
- Supports good bone density, working in tandem with oestrogen

As you work through this chapter, you'll become acquainted with these stages of hormonal maturity. Take note of where you currently sit within this hormonal timeframe:

PRE-MENOPAUSE
From early teenage life when periods begin to around 40 years of age.

PERI-MENOPAUSE
This is where hormones begin to change, progesterone production falters but oestrogen is still pumping.

MENOPAUSE
Literally, the cessation of bleeding - also called 'the change of life'. This is the interval where periods may start to skip a month. Hot flushes and classic menopause symptoms can come and go.

POST-MENOPAUSE
Once periods have been absent for 12 months and hormonal blood tests indicate a classical menopause pattern of low oestrogen and progesterone, a woman will receive her post-menopausal badge of honour. She is now a truly wise woman of our tribe.

No matter what your age, we encourage you to read through the problems and solutions for each of these phases of womanhood. You will then be able to arm yourself with the tools necessary for a smooth transition through the inevitable hormonal changes of life. These tools will also help you to prepare yourself to mentor the younger women in your life.

Pre-menopause: from maidenhood to babies and beyond

This period encompasses the time from the onset of periods to the completion of the fertile years. Typically this is around the age of 40.

The first time a woman is confronted with the possibility of hormonal imbalance is at 'menarche', the medical term for when a woman has her first period. Teenagers beginning their relationship with monthly menstrual bleeding may be plagued with cyclical symptoms of headaches and heavy period flow. This is the first opportunity for women to experience oestrogen dominance – where oestrogen starts to cycle in response to our innate biological clock, but progesterone is still sleeping.

The body has delicate balancing and feedback cycles to keep the levels of these two hormones 'just right'. Women will pay a price for both too little and too much of either hormone at any age.

MENSTRUATION AND MIGRAINES

Young girls experiencing menstrual migraine can respond well to a safe and simple herbal remedy. The herb Chaste tree, or Vitex 1000mg taken each day before breakfast for three months can promote healthy progesterone levels and iron out the hormonal bumps of puberty in those first few period cycles.

THE MENSTRUAL CYCLE

MENSTRUATION

This is the period when the endometrium
or lining of the uterus sheds over 3-7 days
if there is no pregnancy.

LUTEAL PHASE

This is when the endometrium
(the lining of the uterus) is thick and
prepared to support a pregnancy
or be released in a period.

FOLLICULAR PHASE

This is when several eggs mature inside
small cysts or follicles with the ovary.

OVULATION

This is when an egg is released from the biggest
follicle and travels through the fallopian tube,
where it can be fertilised. If it is not fertilised,
it dissolves in about 24-48 hours.

Your menstrual cycle

Start by familiarising yourself with the ebb and flow of a menstrual cycle in a woman who is thriving and in perfect hormonal alignment. We'll also introduce you to the main players necessary for hormonal harmony.

PHASE ONE

The first half of a natural cycle - the follicular phase - is around two weeks in length. This is when the fertility hormone oestrogen surges to prepare the uterus for a pregnancy by stimulating the thickness of the uterine lining. It is now that you may feel at your peak performance. Oestrogen is a cognitive hormone, and helps with the brain's ability to multi-task and perform cognitively at this time. You should be unaware of any hormonal symptoms at this point in the month - everything is happening behind the scenes.

As oestrogen stimulates the blood flow to the uterus, the lining of the uterus thickens. Oestrogen is still in charge until this half of the cycle is completed. The other fertility hormone, progesterone, sits quietly waiting for a signal from the ovary that the time has come to shine. Just before midcycle, in response to a rising level of the ovarian hormone LH (luteinising hormone), progesterone starts to surge. This slightly raises the body temperature a tiny half a degree from baseline.

As oestrogen levels are peaking, a woman may be become aware of changes in the vaginal mucus to make it more welcoming to sperm. You may see a stretchy, egg-white consistency of fertile mucus in your underwear or when you go to the toilet.

The graph below shows the typical levels of a woman in hormonal balance, when she is in a **Thriving State of Being**.

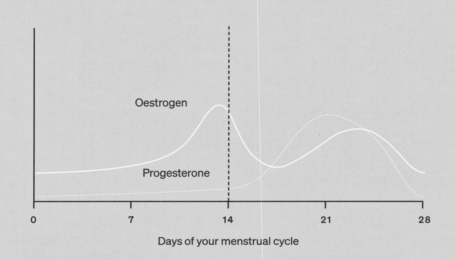

PREGNANCY AND BLEEDING: AN EXPLANATION

Occasionally, just after fertilisation of an egg, an 'implantation bleed' may occur. This can cause a spot of blood to be visible, which may be interpreted as the beginning of an early period bleed rather than the first physical signs of pregnancy. It is perfectly normal. Of course, if you are worried, always contact your GP or gynaecologist for advice and reassurance.

Combining the slight temperature increase with vaginal mucus change is also nature's way of signalling the fertile time immediately ahead. Women can use this information both as a guide to pregnancy planning and a natural form of contraception. Contraception is also made more reliable by the use of a barrier contraceptive such as a diaphragm or condoms during sex.

PHASE TWO

The mid-cycle, or fertile time of the menstrual month is where conception may happen. A healthy egg is released from its sac within the ovary. This sac is lined with an important nest of cells called the corpus luteum. The egg travels down the fallopian tube to enter the uterus. A robust sperm meets the newly released egg, winning the race of survival of the fittest to create a new human. If all the stars are aligned, the fertilised egg will embed in a lusciously thick and nurturing uterine lining. This will be the start of a healthy pregnancy for a woman in a **Thriving State of Being**.

The progesterone hormone continues to rise during this early phase of pregnancy, produced primarily by the corpus luteum until the placenta is ready to take over the job around three months into the pregnancy.

If pregnancy is not a possibility this month, balanced hormones continue to provide a healthy surge of progesterone throughout the second half of the menstrual month. This is called the 'Luteal Phase'.

OVULATION PAIN? HERE'S WHAT TO DO

In general, the ovaries share the job of egg production, alternating from the left to right ovary, month by month. Some women will get pain from the site of the egg release (known as the corpus luteum), if a small amount of fluid has also built up in the buffer zone of the egg. This pain is medically referred to as *Mittelschmerz* (German for 'middle pain'). This pain traditionally occurs every second month, when one ovary is a little slow to do its job to efficiently release the egg. This pain can be severe enough to need analgesics in some women. A herbal preparation containing the herb called Chaste Tree combined with the Cramp Bark herb works well in this scenario.

PHASE THREE

If fertilisation of the released egg does not happen, hormonal signals are sent to the reproductive control centre. These signals will tell your body to complete the menstrual cycle by shedding that month's uterine lining. Your body will then start the preparation process anew after the period bleed has done its job. The period bleed should start cleanly with only a little spotting preceding four to five days of bright red vaginal bleeding. A little cramping on Day 1 and 2 is common, but should be easily settled by simple strategies.

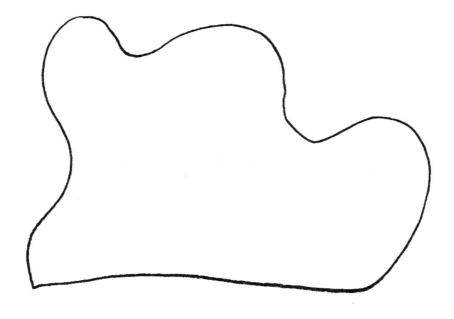

Hysterectomy? Still suffering from monthly cramps? Here's why...

Most women don't realise that period cramps originate predominantly from bowel spasms rather than the uterus. **For some women who have had a hysterectomy, it can be bitterly disappointing to continue to experience a monthly cycle of pain.** This is related to the effect of cramping hormones called prostaglandins which may continue to irritate the smooth muscle of the bowel in the absence of a uterus.

Try this natural solution for mild period cramps. Before reaching for the pharmaceutical options for period pain, try an over-the-counter herbal preparation marketed for irritable bowel symptoms. The product, Iberogast, contains the following herbals: Iberis amara (a bitter candytuft); angelica root; chamomile; caraway fruit; St Mary's thistle; lemon balm; peppermint; greater celandine and liquorice root.

This product has been medically tested in clinical trials and is used in conventional medicine and hospitals for bowel pain and cramping.

Another herbal that works is Cramp Bark. As the traditional name implies, this herb has been used for centuries to help women treat menstrual cramping naturally.

WHAT DOES 'NATURAL' FLOW LOOK AND FEEL LIKE?

Your menstrual flow should be easy to control with pads, tampons or a menstrual cup, changed every four to six hours. A pad designed for overnight use should easily hold the flow for eight hours of normal sleep, with no flooding.

If you ever experience any of the following, it could be a warning sign that your flow is heavier than that of a 'natural' cycle (even if it seems normal for you). Note that Day 1 is defined as the first day of bright red vaginal bleeding.

- You need to change your tampon or menstrual pad more than every three hours on your heavy flow day (usually Day 1 or 2)
- Bright red blood loss lasting for more than five days
- Spotting that continues for more than one day after the end of bright red flow
- Spotting that begins more than one day before the start of bright red bleeding
- Periods that come more frequently than every 26 days
- The presence of blood clots in the toilet or on pads

These signs are red flags for hormonal imbalance, and could lead to iron deficiency and, if left unchecked, anaemia. This can then create a health spiral leading to a Depleted State of Being. If you experience any of these during your menstrual flow, discuss it with your health practitioner and make sure that your iron stores are checked.

Blood tests for iron stores performed just after the end of a period (around Day 8) are more indicative of a depletion. This will be when iron studies are at their lowest and are more likely to coincide with how you feel.

HITTING THE SWEET SPOT WITH IRON – AN ESSENTIAL NUTRIENT

Iron deficiency is the most common nutritional deficiency in the world. Believe it or not, iron is an essential ingredient for over 90 different biochemical processes in the human body. It is a true multi-tasker. When you consider the many important roles iron has to play, it becomes obvious that a deficiency in this vital mineral will have far-reaching effects on health, causing exhaustion but leading ultimately to hormonal havoc, auto-immune disease and depression.

Women frequently present with severe iron deficiency, called *anaemia*. The condition usually develops from many years of low dietary iron intake and is often exacerbated by heavy periods or regular blood donations.

IRON DEFICIENCY PRECEDES ANAEMIA

Women with anaemia will quite often cope unknowingly, until they are particularly stressed with illness or pregnancy.

If the same degree of anaemia that is often discovered in women who are going about their normal daily lives had been caused by an acute major injury, the prescribed treatment would involve hospitalisation and blood transfusion!

Many people are confused about the difference between iron deficiency and anaemia. Immature red blood cells require iron to be converted by the body into a form they can use in order to mature. When fully matured, they will have a very important job to perform. They will become the oxygen-carriers of the body, distributing oxygen from the lungs to every other cell.

Iron deficiency is the first phase towards a decrease in the amount of oxygen-carrying, iron-rich haemoglobin within each red blood cell. As red cells are deprived of their quota of iron, they become contracted and smaller (known in medical terms as becoming microcytic). Anaemia develops when the immature red cells, deprived of their quota of iron, fail to survive their infancy. A formal diagnosis of anaemia is made when there is a consequent and significant decrease in the number of mature red blood cells.

The progression of iron deficiency to anaemia:

NORMAL BLOOD FILM
Plenty of plump, iron-rich
red blood cells.

IRON DEFICIENCY
Same number of cells, but smaller
in size due to low iron, losing some
oxygen-carrying capacity.

**IRON DEFICIENCY
(ANAEMIA)**
Loss of red blood cells –
less in number and much
smaller again, with limited
oxygen-carrying capacity.

Raw iron obtained from food sources has to be converted by the body into a serviceable form of iron called ferritin before it can be used by cells. A severe iron deficiency may still be the cause of extreme tiredness even though raw iron (serum iron) levels are normal or even high.

SYMPTOMS OF IRON DEFICIENCY:
EXHAUSTION
SHORTNESS OF BREATH ON EXERTION
MUSCLE ACHE AND CRAMPS
RAPID PULSE AND HEART PALPITATIONS
INCREASED ANXIETY
BRAIN FOG
POOR MEMORY AND CONCENTRATION
HEADACHES
DEPRESSION
INCREASE IN THE NUMBER OF INFECTIONS

Women can be suffering a severe iron deficiency in spite of being given the all-clear from their doctor. We now know this is because the common blood test done for iron is not indicative of the true usable iron in red cells and tissues. To completely rule out iron deficiency, the following four tests are needed:

SERUM IRON
Serum iron is the raw iron absorbed directly from food.

TOTAL IRON-BINDING CAPACITY
This capacity will be increased above reference range as a result of iron deficiency because the body will attempt to adapt and bind any remaining iron it has available to it.

TRANSFERRIN SATURATION
In layman's terms, this is the percentage of the red blood cell that has actually been saturated with iron (apologies to science graduates for this oversimplification of a complex term).

SERUM FERRITIN

This test reveals the usable iron reserves of the body.

Iron deficiency may create a vicious cycle as it creates a biochemical stress on your body. This can indirectly drive oestrogen dominance and create a heavier blood loss in the next menstrual month.

DONATING YOUR BLOOD

Unfortunately, when you give blood, they will only screen you for anaemia, not for pre-anaemic levels of iron deficiency. Women in particular may be severely iron deficient and still pass the test for blood donor qualification. If you have ticked the warning signs for heavy menstrual loss, make sure to check full iron studies before you donate blood.

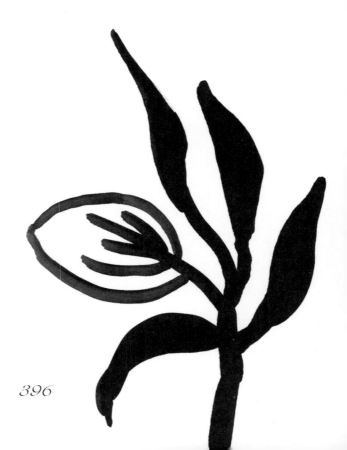

THE ORAL CONTRACEPTIVE PILL

The oral contraceptive pill (commonly known as the Pill) has been available to women since the 1960s. At that time there were very few options available to women who wished to take control of their reproductive choices.

The Pill continues to be a common contraceptive choice for women. There are some women who are prescribed the Pill because of heavy bleeding or flooding during their period. These women will, by definition, be in a Depleted State of Being. For some, the choice of the Pill is the right one to help them buy some time to put in place the plans outlined on page 407. For others, the lifestyle and more natural support outlined in this book will lead to a thriving state of hormonal harmony without the need for powerful prescription medication. Young women who have been counselled through the risks/benefits analysis of the Pill for contraception will make the right choice for their unique circumstances.

WHY THE PILL MAY BE UNHELPFUL

This natural ebb and flow of monthly hormonal changes are completely hijacked by the oral contraceptive pill. The levels of oestrogen and progesterone-mimicking hormones are dictated by the brand of the pill. The vaginal bleeding that happens every month on the pill is more correctly called a 'withdrawal bleed', rather than a true period. This bleed is triggered when a woman abruptly stops the high-level hormonal pills and starts the inactive or sugar pills. Any hormonal symptom while taking the oral contraceptive pill is a side effect of that brand of pill, not a natural symptom of innate hormonal imbalance. Trialling different pill combinations can help you find the best long-term brand that suits you. This is best tackled with the help of a doctor with a special interest in women's reproductive health.

WHEN THINGS GO WRONG - HORMONAL DISTRESS

The graph below is typical of a woman with premenstrual symptoms: irritability, bloating, fluid retention, breast tenderness and tiredness. Her periods may come more frequently than once a month, and will be heavier than those of young women in a **Thriving State of Being**.

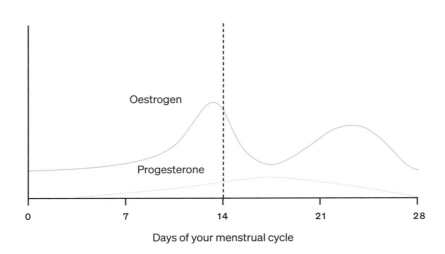

Days of your menstrual cycle

Welcome to the not-so-pleasant world of oestrogen dominance. Oestrogen takes the lead through the menstrual month, but in fact the actual amount of oestrogen produced is just about normal – it is the progesterone that fails to fill its essential role in the second half of this dance and oestrogen dominates the full menstrual month. This is the hormonal scenario of Premenstrual Syndrome, or PMS. The symptoms of PMS are identical to the symptoms of low progesterone in the luteal phase (second half) of the menstrual cycle.

SYMPTOMS OF LOW PROGESTERONE

IRRITABILITY

MIGRAINE

HEADACHES

LOSS OF LIBIDO

DEPRESSION

BACKACHE

FLUID RETENTION

BLOATING

FATIGUE

WEIGHT GAIN

MOOD SWINGS

SORE AND/OR LUMPY BREASTS

A low progesterone level in the luteal phase means that oestrogen dominates the full four weeks of a menstrual month. In doing this, the lining of the uterus continues to thicken well beyond the time needed for healthy pregnancy preparation, creating a much heavier menstrual loss. The lack of hormonal signals (a sharp drop in progesterone around day 27 to 28) and a thicker-than-average uterine lining means that pre-period spotting is commonplace. This spotting can sometimes start a full week before the true period and will contribute to an increased overall blood loss.

Athletes take note!

Karen says: 'As a part of my medical practice, I have been fortunate to care for some of the world's best female athletes in endurance sports, the marathon and triathlon arenas. These young women pay a particularly high price in hormonal balance to achieve their personal goals in their sporting careers.

'I remember one woman coming to see me for advice on how to manage her increasingly heavy periods that would impact her performance if peaking for an important event. She recounted her coach's solution when she mentioned to him that her periods were becoming a problem. He told her: "If you're still having periods then you obviously aren't training hard enough."

'This comment was alarming on so many levels. Fortunately, we began to tackle the issue of hormonal balance in a more constructive and balanced way.'

Although elite athletes carry a unique burden of hormonal challenges, the same situation can be triggered in women who are attempting to embark on new and healthy habits and therefore, unfortunately, reduce healthy fats in their diet. A woman with a low body weight (for example, a BMI below 18) will almost certainly stop having periods, regardless of her athletic ability.

There are several reasons why this happens. Firstly, low body weight triggers ancient pathways of survival. The brain interprets both high stress and low-fat or low calorie intake as a possible drought, famine or war emergency. The emergency centre within the brain signals a stop to the production of the trigger hormones FSH from the brain and LH from the ovary. First progesterone slows, causing erratic and heavier than average periods that come more frequently than the usual 28 days. Eventually oestrogen production stops. As the menstrual cycle goes into hibernation, periods disappear.

HORMONES AND CHOLESTEROL

The 'grandmother' of all sex hormones, both male and female, is *cholesterol*. It provides the design and building blocks for their construction as it also does for the anti-inflammatory hormone, *pregnenolone*. Note the striking similarity between the hormones shown in the illustration below, all derived from the cholesterol framework.

CHOLESTEROL FRAMEWORK

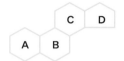

The cholesterol unit is the hormonal building block
for the following hormones:

OUR STRESS HORMONE

Cortisol

OUR ANTI-FLAMMATORY HORMONE

OUR SEX HORMONES

Progesterone

Oestrogen

Testosterone

Efforts to lower levels in order to avert heart disease in low-risk women may create unnecessary hormone chaos. Interfering with the anti-inflammatory pathways can increase vulnerability to the autoimmune diseases. This can result from increased inflammatory pathways. Taking everything into consideration, striking a balance with cholesterol levels obviously has its merits.

OESTROGEN DOMINANCE

By now you should have a handle on what it's like to experience oestrogen dominance due to a low progesterone. Maybe you have ticked a lot of the symptoms listed in the *low progesterone* box. But what happens if the oestrogen message is also amplified?

Oestrogen dominance can take various forms. While it is not specifically a 'medical disease', it can have devastating effects on personal health and increase the risk of oestrogen-responsive cancers like uterine and breast cancer. In common PMS issues, the problem is fundamentally that low progesterone gives oestrogen the control by default. If oestrogen is also raised even modestly above natural levels, the hormonal consequences are ramped up and we see the effect in complex medical conditions such as polycystic ovarian syndrome (PCOS) and Premenstrual Dysphoric Disorder, or PMDD.

Excessive oestrogen challenges the biochemical pathways of hormone recycling. The end result can be a build-up of nasty compounds called DNA adducts. These home-made bad guys insert themselves into the genetic code of cells undergoing division during cell replenishment and growth. Breast tissue is very sensitive to these naturally occurring DNA adducts. The unhealthy message that is coded into the DNA of the new breast cell can eventually lead to a diagnosis of cancer.

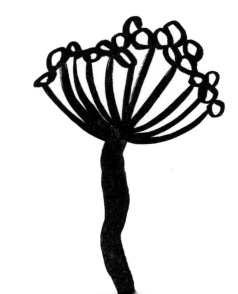

A NOTE ON PCOS (POLYCYSTIC OVARIAN SYNDROME)

Women diagnosed with PCOS may have the following hormonal issues to deal with:

- high oestrogen - oestrogen dominance
- high androgens (male hormones) - leading to acne and weight gain
- increased baseline stress hormones (in particular, cortisol)
- absent periods - because of complex hormonal and adrenal impairment
- insulin resistance
- weight gain

Take this mini-audit on PCOS

- O Are you missing periods for no reason?
- O Is your skin breaking out?
- O Are you struggling with your weight?
- O Do you have a problem with excess body hair?
- O Do you crave sugar and carbs?

PCOS is a complex medical condition and is beyond the scope of this book. If you answered 'yes' to any of these above questions, you'll find a link to solutions in the Resources section. Please read through these and bring your symptoms to the attention of your doctor.

PREMENSTRUAL DYSPHORIC DISORDER (PMDD)

Over the past decade, severe premenstrual symptoms have now become medically recognised as Premenstrual Dysphoric Disorder, or PMDD. This is a complex hormonal disorder and affects the interplay between reproductive hormones and nervous system hormones like serotonin and GABA. The symptoms of PMS are then amplified to screaming levels. Oestrogen levels will often be well above reference range for the midcycle time, but dramatic changes in both oestrogen and progesterone are the hallmarks of PMDD. The only reprieve from symptoms is the few days around the end of period time.

SYMPTOMS OF PMDD CAN INCLUDE:

- severe mood swings with irritability and tears
- depression
- suicidal thoughts
- intense anger and aggression
- sensitivity to rejection
- fatigue
- changes in appetite
- sleep disturbance (either insomnia or excessive sleepiness)
- fluid retention
- breast and pelvic pain and congestion

The number of women ticking the boxes for PMDD is rising. There is firm evidence that the oestrogen-mimicking chemicals play a major role in this increasingly common problem in young women and can be a form of extreme oestrogen dominance. Measurement of natural oestrogens may be normal in this instance, as the oestrogen mimics are not measured on a routine hormonal blood test. If you tick the symptom listed above, pay particular attention to the solutions on page 407 and 408. Connect with an experienced practitioner in Women's Health to guide you further, as medication may provide a welcome reprieve from severe symptoms while you implement the solutions in this chapter.

THE HORMONAL HAVOC OF PERIMENOPAUSE

Don't let oestrogen dominance hijack your 40s. Although a flattening of the progesterone production can occur at any age, women entering their 40s are more vulnerable to this pattern of hormonal imbalance. This is referred to as perimenopause, where the nurturing progesterone erratically fails to deliver its message in the second half of the menstrual cycle, leaving the demon hormone oestrogen in charge for the whole month.

Overtraining, low body weight or poor dietary fat intake will affect women of all ages, but the effects are more brutal as we enter perimenopause.

A typical woman in perimenopause will still be having periods. The periods are often heavier than normal and may go for a day or two longer than the typical four- to five-day bleed. A woman in perimenopause may be late with her period, and often complains of irritability, bloating, fluid retention and tiredness. These are all symptoms of low progesterone. Added to this will be a touch of menopausal symptoms as oestrogen surges one month and plunges the next. In fact, this woman will only briefly feel 'normal' for three to four days after the end of her period.

With the failure of the healthy progesterone surge at midcycle, the nightmare begins again for herself, her family and her workmates. The flatter the response of the progesterone hormone in the second half of the cycle, the more severe the symptoms. The more fluctuating the oestrogen levels, the more likelihood of flushing and brain fog.

Perimenopause is a confusing term that encompasses hormonal changes that can start a decade or more before true menopause. It is vital to understand how hormonal balance can begin to change well before periods stop completely and we enter the 'change of life' that doctors call menopause. True menopause occurs when the oestrogen hormones drop dramatically, heralding the cessation of period bleeding.

A woman in perimenopause may visit her doctor, who will check for classical menopause by looking for low oestrogen. If a hormonal check is not done in the second half of the cycle, where the progesterone surge should ideally occur, then the normal oestrogen on her blood test will be falsely reassuring.

At this perimenopausal stage in life, the oestrogen is still plentiful. A woman in this situation is often told that her hormones are 'normal', that she is not in menopause. As the result of badly timed hormonal checks, many women leave their doctor's surgery with a prescription for antidepressants rather than advice for hormonal wellness.

To diagnose perimenopause, make sure to have a hormonal blood test around day 18 to 22 of the menstrual month or when your symptoms are at their worst. This will confirm a low progesterone and confirm adequate oestrogen levels that don't qualify for a diagnosis of 'menopause.' The brain hormone FSH should also be within the normal range in perimenopause. Women in a Depleted State of Being are more likely to have symptoms of low progesterone in perimenopause, and perimenopause will produce hormonal stress that can push women into this state – a vicious cycle.

PERIMENOPAUSE: HOW TO ACHIEVE HORMONAL BALANCE

Hormonal balance is achieved by ensuring adequate cholesterol levels, low stress levels and addressing any nutrient deficiencies like iron, zinc and B vitamins essential to make good hormone levels.

Stress will also affect the way a body makes hormones. Apart from the obvious stresses of illness and a pressured lifestyle, nutritional deficiencies can also stress your body.

The hormonal imbalance of perimenopause also contributes to iron deficiency through heavier bleeding; iron deficiency is also a common cause of heavy periods. An unfortunate Catch-22 to say the least!

SOLUTIONS TO THE HORMONAL HAVOC OF PERIMENOPAUSE

1 **Good bowel health**: the bowel is your nutrient extraction factory and low nutrient levels will affect hormone production.

2 **Quality counts**: ensure adequate amounts of good-quality fats and oils are in your diet. Natural fats and oils are found in nuts, seeds, advocado and oily fish such as sardines and salmon.

3 **Increase cruciferous vegetables**: these include broccoli, Brussels sprouts, cabbage and cauliflower. Broccoli and broccolini are superfoods when it comes to ironing out hormonal imbalance as they provide the body with Sulforaphane. Sulforaphane increases the efficiency of the genes responsible for oestrogen metabolic pathways. Unlike the other members of the cruciferous family, broccoli does *not* contain progoitrin and cannot impact on thyroid health.

4 **Support liver health**: liver loaders like alcohol, caffeine and sugar will distract the liver from its job as a hormone modulator, and make perimenopause symptoms worse. Consider doing a short liver cleanse or detox (see page 133 for our Liver Support Guide).

HERBS TO HELP YOUR HORMONES

- Chaste tree herb – 500-1000mg taken each morning during the full menstrual month can support healthy progesterone levels.

- Evening Primrose oil can soothe painful swollen breasts. Take a dose of 1000mg three times daily.

- St John's Wort herb - 1000mg daily can reduce symptoms of low mood or irritability. Note that St John's Wort should not be taken with any anti-depressant medication, and can interfere with other pharmaceutical drugs. Check with your pharmacist before taking.

- Bio-identical progesterone: consider wild yam derived, bioidentical, natural progesterone in a transdermal cream, oral capsule or troche (sublingual lozenge). This is available on prescription from a doctor with a special interest in bio-identical hormone support.

VITAMINS AND MINERALS FOR HORMONE BALANCE

- Vitamin B6: 50 to 100mg daily is a natural fluid releaser/diuretic.

- Magnesium: 300mg daily can reduce muscle tension.

- Sulforaphane supplement: this well-credentialled, broccoli-derived natural product can have positive impact on the gene pathways responsible for oestrogen, vitamin D, inflammation and detoxification. Its track record is impressive.

DON'T LET MENOPAUSE SABOTAGE WELLNESS

Why is it that a woman can suddenly resemble an overboiling radiator on even the coldest of days? Why does she have to endure the embarrassment of a flushed, moisture-laden face at the most inappropriate times? Why does she have to change sweat-soaked sheets every morning and don a new outfit every few hours?

Menopause will often hit a woman when she's at a transition time with family and work demands. These external pressures can make it very challenging to smoothly walk through the menopause door. Sleep can be sabotaged due to night sweats or high stress hormones.

In this transition period, oestrogen levels can fluctuate dramatically from month to month. Blood tests will show a rise in the brain hormone FSH, and a lower than expected oestrogen. Expect this to last for around 12 months, but it could last anywhere from just one month to several years in some women.

SOLUTIONS FOR HORMONAL HARMONY IN MENOPAUSE

This transition period can be challenging for many women, with the fluctuation of hormones from one month to the next. Once hormones have settled into their postmenopausal baseline, symptoms diminish and should only recur if one of the **Five Pillars of Wellness** are out of balance.

Stress can create a domino effect on the hormonal symptoms of menopause. Any stress on the body will raise both cortisol and adrenaline hormones. See our chapters on Stress Resilience (Chapter 6, 7 and 8) for solutions to support a smooth transition through menopause.

KEEP YOUR STRESS LEVELS UNDER CONTROL

Cortisol – the stress hormone – is a catabolic hormone, meaning it breaks down tissue and in particular, muscle mass. This can impact bone density and strength, potentially increasing the risk of falls.

Stress will impact sleep as it drives cortisol levels higher. Withania somnifera (also known as Ashwagandha, winter cherry or Indian ginseng) is an adrenal support herb that can buffer the effect of cortisol. Look for a product that provides around 1000mg of withania dried herb per tablet. The usual dose is between three and six tabs daily. Review Chapter 9 to make sure your sleep strategies are well in place before menopause hits.

Anything that puts a chemical load on the liver will compromise the body's ability to gain good hormonal balance through menopause. Alcohol, high sugar diets, caffeine and even simple medications such as paracetamol are all liver loaders. Alcohol will take direct aim at the hot flush control button and activate it every time. Nurturing liver health means a much smoother rite of passage through menopause, with less impact on quality of sleep.

WHEN SHOULD YOU EXPERIENCE MENOPAUSE?

Natural menopause is expected between the ages of 48 and 54, although new research has linked early menopause with a woman's lifetime exposure to toxic 'forever' chemicals called PFAFS. These chemicals accumulate over decades as your body is unable to eliminate them. The research showed that women who measured in the highest 25 per cent of total body burden of these chemicals had reset their biological clock and brought their natural menopause forward a staggering two years.

Review Chapter 10 to minimise your exposure to these hormonally horrible chemicals.

HERBAL SOLUTIONS FOR HOT FLUSHES AND NIGHT SWEATS

Herbal solutions are worth considering if you're experiencing hot flushes and night sweats as a first option before going to your doctor. Red Clover in particular deserves honourable mention. The active ingredients in Red Clover are the isoflavones. A dose of 80mg is needed to control hot flushes. At 40mg the isoflavones in Red Clover have been shown to support bone density. Black Cohosh has also been used traditionally for hot flushes. Rarely, a woman may have side effects from this product, including liver inflammation.

If menopause symptoms are intolerable, discuss the pros and cons of bioidentical hormone options versus standard Hormone Replacement Therapy (HRT) with an integrative doctor who has a special interest in female health. It is important to consider both risks and benefits of both options. Formal HRT is back in fashion with the medical profession. If the dose is kept low and a transdermal application is used – a patch or cream – the impact of that particular hormone on the liver can be minimised. If the use is limited to less than 12 months, the breast cancer risk associated with the oestrogen component of HRT is reduced.

Common sense and balance is king when it comes to optimal wellness. For some, it may be necessary to pull back on extreme training to gain hormonal balance. Alternate heavy training days with more gentle movement activities to rediscover hormonal harmony that every woman deserves. Review Chapter 5 and make sure you hit your 'sweet spot' with exercise.

Listen to your body as it makes the transition through perimenopause to post-menopausal wellness and embrace, rather than fight against, the changes in your body.

Always start with the gentle hormonal supports. Although lifestyle choices like limiting alcohol are more socially challenging, they provide a safer option that will domino into benefits beyond hormonal harmony.

POST-MENOPAUSE AND BALANCE

A natural post-menopause state in a thriving woman should be hormonally as carefree as childhood. Consistently low levels of the two fertility hormones, oestrogen and progesterone, tick over, providing adequate hormonal support for good cognition and bone density support into post-menopausal life.

Oestrogen levels are the same, from day to day, week to week, month to month. Lack of dramatic fluctuations in oestrogen allows a healthy post-menopausal woman to breeze through the day and night without a hot flush. Levels of oestrogen in blood tests should be steady, around 40 to 100.

For those who have a concern about ovarian cancer due to family history, or a history of endometriosis (this raises ovarian cancer risk), a baseline test for a tumour-marker called Cancer Antigen 125 (or Ca 125 for short) may be useful. These tests may not qualify for a government rebate through Medicare, but can be a useful tool as a baseline for sorting out any potential pelvic symptoms into the future.

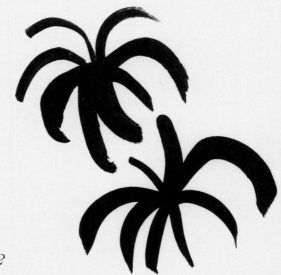

CASE STUDY | DR KAREN

Fiona

Fiona was a well woman who had just celebrate her 60th birthday. She came in complaining of a vague 'feeling of something not right' in her lower abdomen. She had breezed through menopause without the need for hormone replacement therapy, maintaining a healthy body weight and exercising regularly. In fact, she ticked all the boxes of a thriving woman. Her only past health issue related to her pelvis was a laparoscopy (keyhole surgery) for investigation of infertility in her late 20s, where a small patch of endometriosis was removed. She had gone on to have two healthy pregnancies and her children were now thriving adults.

Her mother had undergone a hysterectomy and removal of all but a tiny amount of one ovary at the age of 34 for severe endometriosis but was now in her mid-80s and well.

I felt reassured when her pelvic examination was completely normal, but sent her for blood and urine tests as a starting point for investigating her symptoms. She had a baseline Ca 125 (**Cancer antigen 125** is a protein found in ovarian cancer cells) done in her early 50s. The result was then reassuringly low at 9 units/ml.

The Ca125 tumour marker came back at 29 (the reference range is >35 units/ml). Even though this was still within the acceptable range, this raised my index of suspicion as it was over triple her baseline from eight years previously.

Her pelvic ultrasound was done in the following week, and confirmed a small mass attached to her right ovary. A referral to a local gynaecologist resulted in prompt keyhole surgery and the unexpected finding of an ovarian cancer. Despite this sinister diagnosis, we were relieved that the cancer was at Stage 1A (cancer is in one ovary or fallopian tube, but not on the outer surface), and no further active treatment was required. Within six weeks of her surgery, a repeat Ca125 reading was at 10, where it has remained for the last four years. Fiona remains well.

SOLUTIONS FOR A THRIVING MENOPAUSE

1 **Reduce night sweats**: the return of familiar but mild night sweats associated with times of celebration and a couple of glasses of alcohol, can be tempered by a pre-celebratory dose of the herbal St Mary's thistle and a good multi B vitamin.

2 **Improve lubrication**: a dash of organic coconut oil applied vaginally after a shower should support comfortable love-making for both partners.

3 **Stay on top of your health checks**: keep track of routine health checks and follow your doctor's advice on regular breast screening and pap smears.

4 **Take bone density seriously**: support bone density by adhering to the **Five Pillars of Wellness**. If bone density has been flagged as sub-optimal, the solutions on the following pages should be considered.

THE IMPORTANCE OF VITAMIN D

Ensure that you have adequate vitamin D and make sure to re-check bone density scores at regular intervals. Please note that studies show accelerated bone loss in women whose vitamin D sits below 75 nmol/litre (for women in the US this equates to 30 ng/ml). Women who carry gene variants on their vitamin D receptors will also need higher vitamin D levels to support the movement of vitamin D into the cells of the body, including the bone builder cells called osteoblasts.

When we consider all aspects of vitamin D pathways and importance in the body, it's advised to maintain levels between 80 and 180 nmol/litre. Those with vitamin D gene variations that impair the efficiency of any of these pathways need to stay above 100 nmol/litre. More than 180 is unnecessary if supplementing.

VITAMIN D AND ATHLETES

Karen says: 'The elite triathletes under my care never need vitamin D supplementation – they are, by definition, leading an outdoor life training for their chosen field of sporting excellence. The highest naturally occurring level was 180 nmol/litres in a world champion tri-athlete. In my world, these readings are a more reliable indicator of ideal vitamin D levels than any statistical averaging of "normal population levels" in a world where very few of us lead a natural, outdoor life.'

VITAMIN K

Vitamin K is a good companion to vitamin D as a bone support nutrient. Traditional dried fruits like raisins, prunes and dates are high in vitamin K, along with the bone-building nutrients of manganese, boron and magnesium.

Some questions answered

Q: How much exercise do you need for strong bones?

A: The answer to this may surprise you. Research conducted in 2017 in the UK showed that as little as one to two minutes of running per day can improve bone density scores by four per cent. In fact, women who commit to short bursts of high-intense activity score better than those training for marathons.

This is great news for all time-poor women who want to remain strong and age well. Keep moving, walk often, run sometimes and add some strength training to support good muscle mass. If bone density is low, make sure to do the risk/benefit analysis with your doctor if discussing medication to reduce the risk of bone fractures.

Movement activities like Pilates can solve those pelvic floor bladder control issues, along with a prescription for the natural form of oestrogen called estriol (marketed as Ovestin in Australia and New Zealand).

HOW TO APPLY VAGINAL CREAM

Throw the applicator away when you fill your prescription for Estriol (used to relieve vaginal dryness, itching or irritation associated with the menopause). Instead, apply a centimetre of cream with your finger, three times weekly just after showering. Sweep it around the vulva area (darker skin) and into the vagina as comfortably as you need. Be generous with the cream application around the bladder opening to give maximum support for bladder leakage.

DON'T IGNORE HEART HEALTH

Implementing the solutions in this book will generically support wellbeing, including heart and brain health. Cardiovascular disease is often overlooked in older women. Don't become a statistic. Make sure to tick off the following heart-health checks.:

✓ Make sure that blood pressure readings are nicely within the healthy range: **100 to 129 systolic** - the top number that represents the pressure in the arteries as the heart is pumping; **55 to 84 diastolic** - the resting pressure in between heartbeats.

✓ Have a baseline heart tracing (electrocardiograph or ECG) at your local health clinic.

✓ Get a coronary artery calcium score. This test is recommended for women at the age of 60, or earlier for smokers, ex-smokers and those with a strong family history of heart attack or stroke. This test takes an indirect look at the health of the coronary arteries and can pick up a potential problem up to a decade before changes lead to a heart attack (myocardial infarct). A non-contrast scan is the radiation equivalent of around four standard chest X-rays and can help with the risk/benefit analysis of cholesterol-lowering medication.

Going forward...

The hormonal journey from teenage years through to menopause can be challenging. Regardless of age, existing health issues or hormones, your biochemistry functions on ancient pathways of survival are programmed to do their best to promote good health and longevity. Adopt the solutions based on the **Five Pillars of Wellness**, along with soulful movement, laughter and great company to contribute to a thriving, balanced hormonal State of Being in this modern world.

New research in genetics puts another layer on this complex issue. Hormonal imbalance is exaggerated and harder to remedy in women who carry genetic variations that affect the efficiency of oestrogen metabolic pathways. Turn to Chapter 12 to read about Nutrigenomics and the role they play in determining the risks and benefits of menopausal management with the oestrogen hormone.

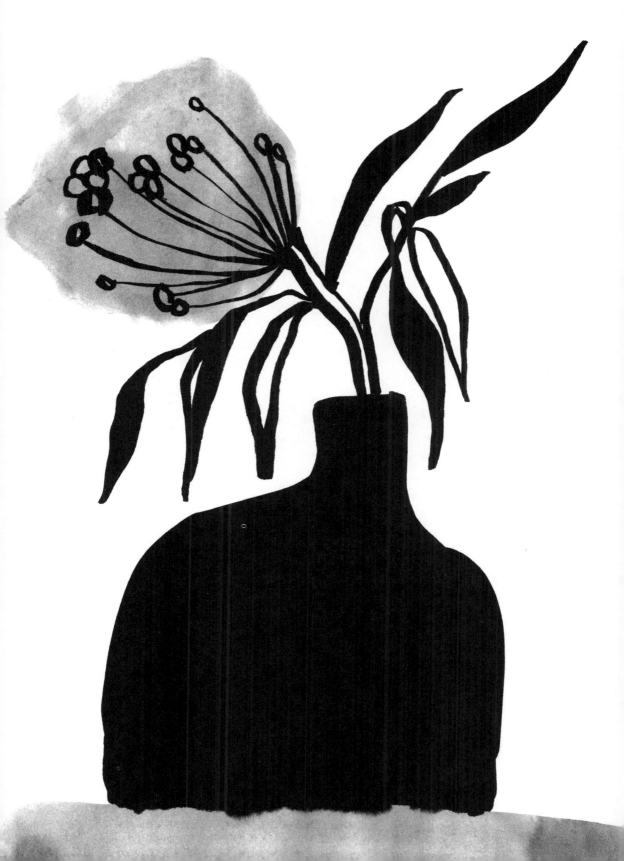

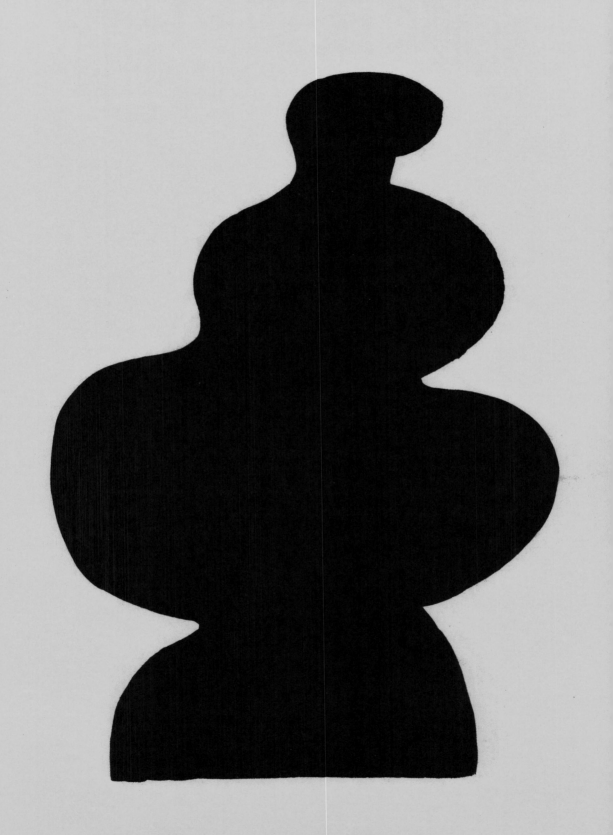

12.
NUTRIGENOMICS

**HOW GENES COMMUNICATE WITH YOUR FOOD,
YOUR ENVIRONMENT AND YOUR BODY**

Genes are
like the story,
and DNA is the
language that
the story is
written in.

SAM KEAN

GENETICS 101 – THE FIRST STEP

The discovery of DNA in 1953 gave the world an understanding of how our ancestors passed on their genetic influences through generations.

The complete DNA library for creating and maintaining the entire human body is stored in the centre (the nucleus) of each and every cell in your body.

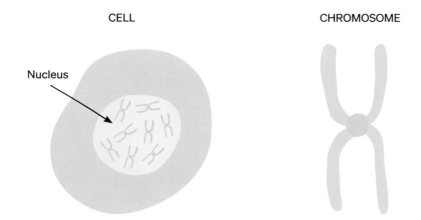

At the moment of your conception, you are blessed with the two complete manuals of 'how to build and maintain a human'. These manuals contain 22 pairs of nearly identical chapters, scientifically known as chromosome pairs. One arm of each chromosome pair comes from your mother, the other from your father. You also have an additional two chromosomes that determines whether you are male (XY) or female (XX) – these are called the x and y chromosomes.

HUMAN KARYOTYPE

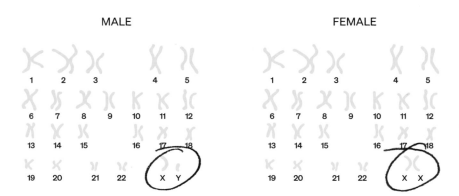

One arm of the chromosome contains a complete genetic code for all body functions from our mother. The other arm from your father's side codes for exactly the same processes but with a slightly different instruction book. Think of this as two complete 'recipes for building a human'. As with all recipes, there are individual differences that may make one 'recipe' an award-winning version compared to a mediocre alternative.

When the sperm and egg combine, both versions of complete recipe books are embedded in your very first cell of your body at the moment of conception. These coded messages use building blocks called nucleotides and deliver Morse code-like instructions on everything that happens in your body.

Your clever cells will select which recipes are appropriate in their unique role to your wellbeing: bone cells read how to make and maintain healthy bone tissue throughout your life; liver cells get on with the job of building new tissue, helping with digestion and making enzymes for your body's detox biochemical pathways, among its many other incredible tasks.

Your body innately chooses which recipe to read – your mother's or father's – as it goes about the job of building and maintaining body structure and making sure that your body functions and thrives from birth onward.

Subtle differences in gene recipes for specific enzymes encoded in our DNA can alter the efficiency of a gene to create its intended end product.

ENZYMES AND DETOXIFICATION

Let's explore this concept of variations from one person to another by looking at genes that code for your detox enzymes. We all have different ancestry based on the area of origin of our family. The majority of your ancestral tribe members will share a common recipe for producing detox enzymes. A minority of people with your ancestral background will have inherited, and use, a slightly different recipe (the gene variation). The commonly available recipe, used by the majority of your genetic tribe, may be the best possible version for this task: making an efficient liver enzyme and giving your body more enzymes to do the job. The less common recipe may slow production lines down or give you less efficient (think lazy) enzymes that makes the hangover headache after a night of celebration much harder to bear. This less-efficient recipe for these enzymes will also result in the slower removal of nasty chemicals, toxins and the by-products of your food digestion process.

The more sluggish gene activity doesn't really matter if we don't give the liver enzymes a challenging job to do - each recipe will be sufficient to do its day job well. But when the liver is challenged to ramp up production, or work overtime to remove the toxic by-products of alcohol from that celebratory night out, the genetic differences in efficiency will become clear.

In women this plays out in a choice that our incredible body must make, in that moment, between two options.

OPTION A

Removing a dangerous toxin like the aldehyde poison from alcohol
as it is processed out of the body.

OPTION B

Do its day job and recycle healthy oestrogen to flow back
to blood vessels and brain cells.

The choice is always **Option A**. In this scenario, a menopausal woman who carries less efficient recipes for making lots of great detox liver enzymes will pay the price in hormonal imbalance, hot flushes and a sleepless night under the detox stress of alcohol.

Early discoveries and genetic research suggested that we may be a victim of our genes, sitting on a genetic time bomb of sorts. It was assumed that a person's DNA firmly set their destiny toward the chronic disease embedded in their family's DNA. It was widely believed that if your parents had cancer or heart disease, it would be highly likely that the genes would express the disease in you. The discovery of a strong breast cancer link with different versions of single genes - such as the BRCA 1 and 2 - had the effect of delivering a life sentence to some women who carried either one of these genes.

EPIGENETICS AND YOU

Further research unlocking the genetic code has given us more optimism and hope. An evolving field of medicine called **Epigenetics** has created quite a stir in research circles over the last two decades. This science tells us we *do* have influence over our genes. Whilst you are born with a set DNA that does not change in your lifetime, your epigenome controls the expression of each gene in your cells. It has an innate ability to turn genes on and off and comes with a volume controller.

The epigenome is a landscape of ever-changing chemical tags called methyl groups that can tightly wrap genes, making them unreadable. Removing the tags unwraps the genes, making them readable again. Your epigenome gives you some control over gene expression. It is heavily influenced by your lifestyle, the food you choose and the environment you are exposed to, both internally and externally.

MIRROR IMAGE

We learn a lot about genes and epigenetics from the study of identical twins. This is how we started to unravel the complexity of the epigenetic switches for the so-called 'bad' genes.

Essentially, twin siblings have a close-to-identical genetic makeup. They come from the same foetal environment, so they (mostly) have the same nutritional influences in the womb.

If genes on their own manifested disease, then we would expect that both identical twins in any family would be destined to develop the same disease within a reasonable time period. But the reality is, that the chances of both twins being affected by any particular disease is only 10 to 20 per cent over their lifetime. This is a much smaller risk than anyone expected. It suggests that the environment (and the interaction of your genes with your environment) is in the driver's seat when it comes to steering your health one way or the other.

GENES: ON OR OFF

The good news is that the majority of us are born with **good genes turned on**, and **bad genes turned off**.

We know that pollutants, chemicals, and toxins, ingested or absorbed through the lungs and skin can have an influence on your gene expression. This is creating quite a stir as any change in genetic expression also has the potential to be passed on to the next generation.

Stress is detrimental to your health on so many levels, including how your genes are expressed. There is also evidence that toxic relationships in all forms, along with chronic stress, are both major factors in gene expression. The impact of a human being living a life of unmanaged pressure, resulting in ongoing, unrelenting stress is devastating to health.

SOLUTIONS FOR ALL STATES OF BEING

OPTIMISING GENETIC POTENTIAL: THE NEW APPROACH TO HEALTHY AGEING

Women of all ages often ask for specific advice on how to maintain function, both physically and cognitively, as they age. For women over 50 years of age, the question of healthy ageing becomes a prominent feature of our conversation.

As we unravel and study the mystery of our genetic heritage, nature provides clear evidence on how to raise the bar to maintain a thriving state. Some people have been dealt a good genetic hand. These people will age more gracefully. For others, targeting specific biochemical areas in their health and wellbeing biochemical pathways will provide clear benefit.

There are several genes that we now recognise as key players in ageing. The genes that are prominent here are the Klotho gene, the APOE gene cluster and the SIRT family of genes.

THE KLOTHO GENE

The Mayo Clinic discovered the Klotho gene and named it after one of the three Greek mythological beings of fate, Klotho, who spun the thread of life and destiny for every mortal from her spindle.

This gene is highly expressed in the blood, brain, and spine. Think of it as a Master Bio-Clock of cellular ageing. When this gene is disrupted, bad things happen. Seriously bad. Like macular degeneration, arteriosclerosis, osteoporosis, renal failure, insulin resistance and premature ageing.

STRATEGIES TO SUPPORT THE KLOTHO GENE PATHWAY:

One of the main disruptors of Klotho is, not surprisingly, cigarette smoke, including passive smoke inhalation and environmental air pollution. This exposure creates different outcomes depending on the person's genetic landscape. It can drive inflammation leading to increased respiratory infections in some people and alter DNA increasing the risk of lung cancer in others.

PROVEN SOLUTIONS FOR HEALTHY EXPRESSION OF KLOTHO

- Avoid all cigarette smoke and other environmental air pollutants where possible.

- Exercise – but make sure not to exceed your 'sweet spot' with aerobic exercise as over-exercise will drive inflammation and turn Klotho **down.**

- Consider supplements containing the herb Withania to support glutathione pathways in the body. Glutathione is important for gene expression of good detoxification pathways.

- The acidophilus probiotic family – research shows a clear link between healthy gut bacteria and longevity acting through the Klotho gene pathway.

- The mushroom cordyceps – available in supplement form and as a dried herb option for cooking.

THE APOE GENE

The APOE gene family rules cognitive health. A significant gene mutation that can be detected in genetic testing is the APOE-4 gene variation where just a single small protein (a base nucleotide) is substituted for another in the genetic recipe that determines the health of our brain neurons. Substituting this one essential ingredient can dramatically alter the quality of the final product, in this case, a healthy brain cell.

When working efficiently, the APOE gene cluster helps break down the amyloid plaque associated with Alzheimer's Disease. With the APOE-4 mutation, the brain cells are more prone to inflammation leading to plaque build-up on neurons that may lead to late-onset dementia.

Fortunately, this negative mutation of APOE is uncommon in our community (in the Western world) but even the favourable version of this gene can do with a little help to maximise cognition into later life. Research shows that supporting this gene activity can increase lifespan and healthy ageing.

PROVEN SOLUTIONS TO SUPPORT THE APOE GENE PATHWAY

- Increase nuts in your diet, especially walnuts. Nuts are rich in good-quality fatty acids. Our brain cells, or neurons, need these fatty acids to build protective insulation sheaths around each neuron.

- Increase omega-3 intake: oily fish, like salmon, herring and eel, or for vegetarians, choose sea-based algae that are rich in omega-3.

- Ingest anti-inflammatory curcumin – both in supplement form and by consuming natural turmeric found in the pantry.

- Use olive oil – a brain superfood.

- Increase manganese-rich foods: seafood, nuts, seeds, and grains.

IS GREEN TEA GOOD FOR YOU?

To answer this question, you must take into consideration the efficiency of an important gene that supports your ability to access the healthy antioxidant in green tea and concentrated green tea extracts like Matcha, that can support brain health in some people.

The COMT gene pathway (officially known as Catechol O Methyl Transferase) is a major player in the body's ability to access and process the specific green tea antioxidants, the catechins and epigallocatechin gallate (EGCG). Can you see a correlation between the names of these antioxidants and the COMT gene? An efficient COMT enzyme is essential for safe access and processing of these specific antioxidants. Those who have inherited a COMT gene variation called the AA allele will struggle to safely break green tea down. This gene variation slows the efficiency of pathways that help process the catechins and pushes these potentially great antioxidants into a dangerous toxic pathway. This can result in catastrophic kidney and liver failure for some people who take high dose green tea extracts or consume more than six to eight green teas per day.

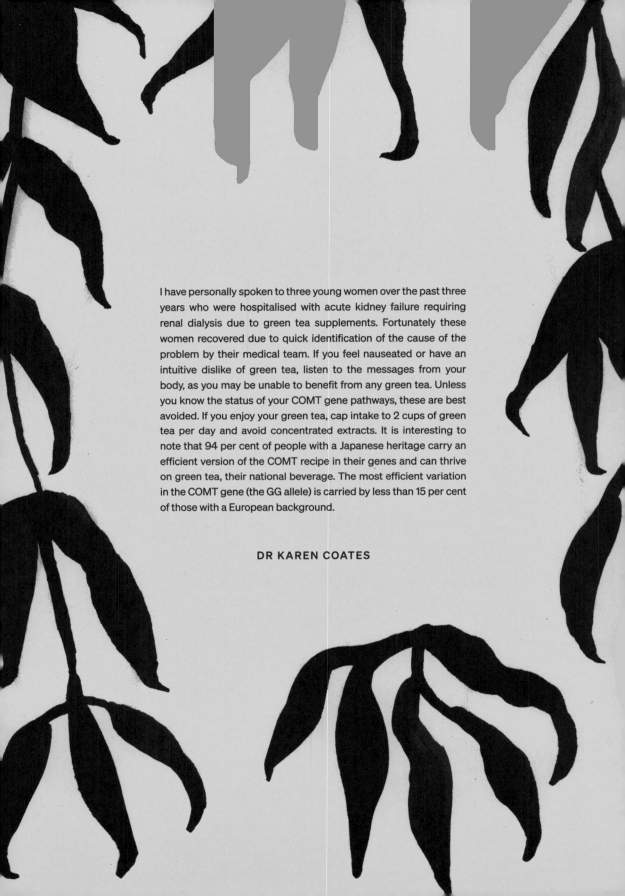

I have personally spoken to three young women over the past three years who were hospitalised with acute kidney failure requiring renal dialysis due to green tea supplements. Fortunately these women recovered due to quick identification of the cause of the problem by their medical team. If you feel nauseated or have an intuitive dislike of green tea, listen to the messages from your body, as you may be unable to benefit from any green tea. Unless you know the status of your COMT gene pathways, these are best avoided. If you enjoy your green tea, cap intake to 2 cups of green tea per day and avoid concentrated extracts. It is interesting to note that 94 per cent of people with a Japanese heritage carry an efficient version of the COMT recipe in their genes and can thrive on green tea, their national beverage. The most efficient variation in the COMT gene (the GG allele) is carried by less than 15 per cent of those with a European background.

DR KAREN COATES

THE SIRT GENE CLUSTER

These genes regulate the production of a group of enzymes called sirtuins, which regulate and slow down the process of ageing. When body cells are put under stress, there are epigenetic changes in genes (on-off switches) that perpetuate cell damage. The sirtuins turn off these inflammatory pathways and keep cells healthy for longer. High activity of the SIRT gene pathway equates to healthier and long lifespan.

PROVEN SOLUTIONS TO SUPPORT THIS GENE PATHWAY

Ensure your diet and lifestyle is rich in the following:

- Zinc (oysters, red meat, pork, nuts and seeds)
- Foods rich in vitamin D, such as oily fish (salmon, anchovies, sardines, herring), organ meats
- Exercise: concentrate on movements such as yoga, Pilates, walking, swimming
- Sunshine
- Cold exposure
- The supplement NAD (from the vitamin B3 family), which can be taken in capsule form or intravenously for a turbo-boost for your cells
- Berberine herb

Remember that your genes are not your destiny, they merely define vulnerabilities.

Implementing support for these pathways, regardless of your genetic landscape, will improve your chances of thriving as you age gracefully.

There is also a clear connection between the health of this good gene and our chromosomes, specifically the tail bit called the telomere. And there's lots of recent information on the importance of maintaining long healthy telomere tails. This brings us back to lifestyle choices.

One of the other telomere disruptors is, not surprisingly, cigarette smoke. This can affect various cells, creating different outcomes depending on the person's genetic landscape:

1   Altering the DNA of the cells (cancer)

2   Changing the inflammation pathways, leading to hypersensitive tissue (asthma, autoimmune disease)

3   Altering immune cell function that protects us from infection

This explains why the lottery of life throws us some lucky individuals who are photographed with a cigar in their mouth and a whiskey in their hands on their 104th birthday. They are the genetically elite of this world, a bit like our elite athletes. Not everyone is so naturally blessed. You don't know whether you are a genetically programmed 'canary' in the mine shaft of our environment. The canaries of this world will get sick first, but given enough exposure to toxins, none of us will be optimally well.

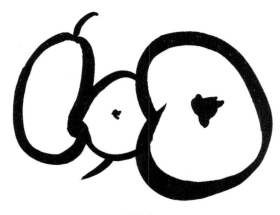

WHAT IS EPIGENETIC CHANGE?

Epigenetic change can occur in a single generation and be passed to future generations. We first saw evidence of the effects of epigenetics by studying the children and grandchildren of Vietnam War veterans, who experienced more than three times the rate of mental health and fertility issues than the average Australian population. This was traced back to the Vets' exposure to multiple chemicals including Agent Orange. This toxin triggered an epigenetic change in the way nervous system hormones were regulated. This change in gene expression was inherited through two generations.

Nutritional medicine has traditionally been overlooked as a main player in health and disease, until gene research forced scientists to return to basic biochemistry. Until the last few years, we had no way of looking at the pathways of chemical reactions that occur constantly in the body, keeping hormone production and energy pathways working efficiently.

Your epigenome affects your gene expression, which in turn affects your health outcomes every day. For heart disease and cancer prevention, the very existence of the epigenome is revolutionary. This is why we are providing you with strong messages to make healthy lifestyle choices. You are literally controlling your genes by how you live every day. The organisation Breast Cancer (**breastcancer.org**) suggests the following preventative measures:

- Maintain a healthy weight
- Exercise regularly
- Limit alcohol
- Eat nutritious food
- Never smoke

These lifestyle choices are vitally important for healthy cells and positive gene expression. It has never been more important to overhaul how you think, feel, move and eat. This is the case for prevention as well as recovery from a disease state.

You literally are the CEO of your own health; your doctors and complementary healthcare practitioners are simply your advisors.

Taking control of your minute-by-minute experience in this life and being mindful of your choices can have an enormous impact on how your body heals and repairs itself.

Globally, healthcare systems are facing major challenges – the world is in the midst of an epidemic of preventable lifestyle diseases. Consequently, even though life expectancy has increased, health expectancy, living in a thriving state of good health, is decreasing.

IS DNA TESTING WORTH IT?

DNA testing for genes that express significant medical diseases have been available for over a decade. As technology improves, the cost of accessing your DNA information has become more affordable. Until recently, genetic information on the drivers of lifestyle disease was devoid of solutions and remained in the hands of academics and researchers. Over the last few years scientists have expanded genetic knowledge to provide information on how it is possible to change the expression of genes to maximise their benefits within an individual. In other words, **your genes are not your destiny**.

We now have access to DNA analysis to check how you scored in the genetic lottery of life by looking at gene clusters that drive these lifestyle diseases. Rather than diagnose disease, this testing shows areas of vulnerability that need more attention as you age.

These 'gene clusters' look at your genetic vulnerability in the following key wellness areas:

- Inflammation
- Cellular detoxification
- Vitamin D pathways
- Methylation pathways and cardiovascular health
- Fat and metabolism
- Hormone processing
- Mood and cognitive function

Before embarking on DNA testing, you should consider the following:

- Does the company providing your DNA analysis have a robust privacy policy and secure database safeguards to protect your sensitive data?
- Companies following best-practice methods will engage firewalls, encryption, intrusion monitoring and passwords to protect all electronic information and testing results. They will also have physical security on their premises with 24-hour monitoring.
- Will the DNA testing affect disclosure for life and disability insurance?

In the US, strong privacy laws protect DNA consumers, and it is illegal for insurance companies to seek DNA results from their customers. In Australia and other countries, the laws are less clear. Some insurance firms are requesting disclosure for new policies. One solution is to have your insurance policies in place prior to embarking on genetic testing.

Are you seeking information on medically significant genes that have direct links to major medical diseases?

For example, consider the BRCA 1 and 2 genes, and the APOE family. This is the area of genetic testing that should remain firmly in the hands of medical specialists. Geneticists have a support network to provide counselling prior to testing, and ongoing support for those who discover that they carry the high-risk form of the gene.

These medical significant genes are 'strongly expressed', meaning that if you carry the high-risk version of the gene, your risk of very serious medical disease is also very high. Carriers of the risk version (or allele) of the BRCA 1 and 2 family have an 80 per cent chance of developing breast or ovarian cancer over their lifetime. Understanding what the results mean for you is an important part of the testing process. You should not receive these results by email from a mail-order do-it-yourself kit.

If you have been tested for these strongly expressed genes and have received news that you carry the high-risk version of the gene, it is even more important for you to take heed of the foundational wellness support contained in this book. Embrace these strategies for wellness, hand-in-hand with your medical options.

CASE STUDY | DR KAREN

Fiona: the sequel

Do you remember Fiona's story from Chapter 11?

One of my special interests is to use DNA tools to provide an insight into the genetic challenges that may affect any of the gene clusters. This becomes the foundation for personalised and targeted programs that can support health goals, provide better information on exercise strategies and rationalise supplements to support wellbeing and healthy ageing.

Research in nutrigenetics highlights several gene clusters that play a role in both breast and ovarian health, outside of the less common BRCA gene family. After Fiona's surgery for her early stage ovarian cancer, she saw a geneticist but elected not to have testing for the BRCA 1 and BRCA 2 genes that can raise risk of gynaecological cancers.

She did proceed with a Health and Wellbeing DNA assessment. Results of Fiona's DNA test looked at the genetic efficiency of her oestrogen and detoxification metabolic pathways. It showed that she would benefit from targeted nutrigenomic support. Implementing these supplements decreased her level of 'catechol' forms of oestrogen that are known to contribute to breast, ovarian and thyroid cancers. Fiona's results also showed red flags on her vitamin D receptor pathways, which made access to optimal vitamin D more difficult for her. We optimised her vitamin D and encouraged her to increase her cruciferous vegetables as these provide a source of sulforaphane. This broccoli derivative can open up the vitamin D receptors and make vitamin D pathways more efficient, regardless of genetic variations in this gene cluster. It has also been well researched for its role in healthy oestrogen metabolism at all ages.

Fiona rediscovered confidence in her body's ability to thrive by implementing these solutions to improve the efficiency of genes that control hormonal balance and healthy oestrogen pathways.

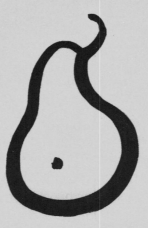

Thank you for taking us into your confidence, and for trusting us with your health issues, worries and concerns. We hope we have helped you as you move towards a healthier, happier and more confident future.

We encourage you to revisit *How to Be Well* into the future, as you (or your family members) face health challenges or when you need a quick reminder of the **Five Pillars of Wellness**.

The first step towards better health begins with you. We trust that with the information we have armed you with, your journey towards a **Thriving State of Being** is just around the corner.

Be well,

DR KAREN COATES AND SHARON KOLKKA

I am the master
of my fate;
I am the captain
of my soul.

WILLIAM ERNEST HENLEY

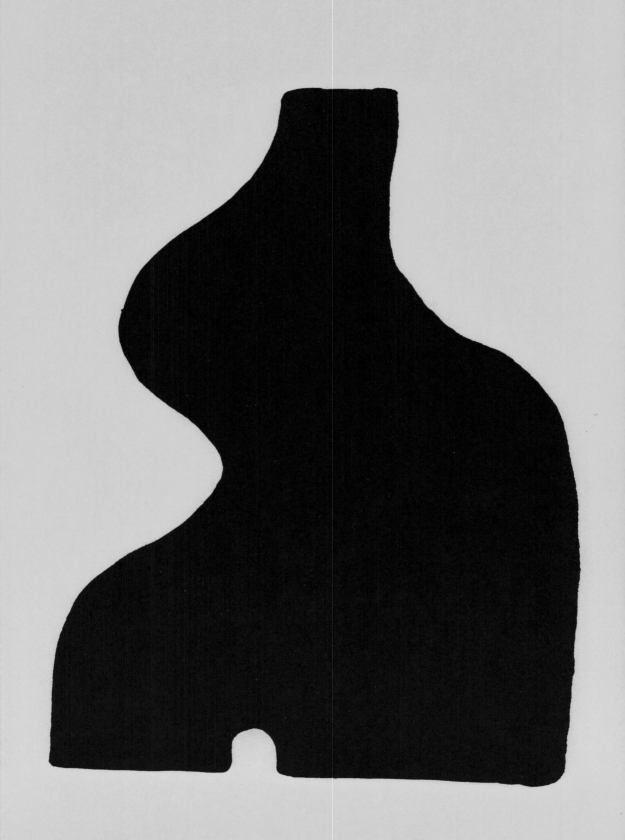

13.
YOUR DAILY HEALTH AND WELLNESS SOLUTIONS

Healthy habits
are learned in
the same way as
unhealthy ones –
through practice.

WAYNE DYER

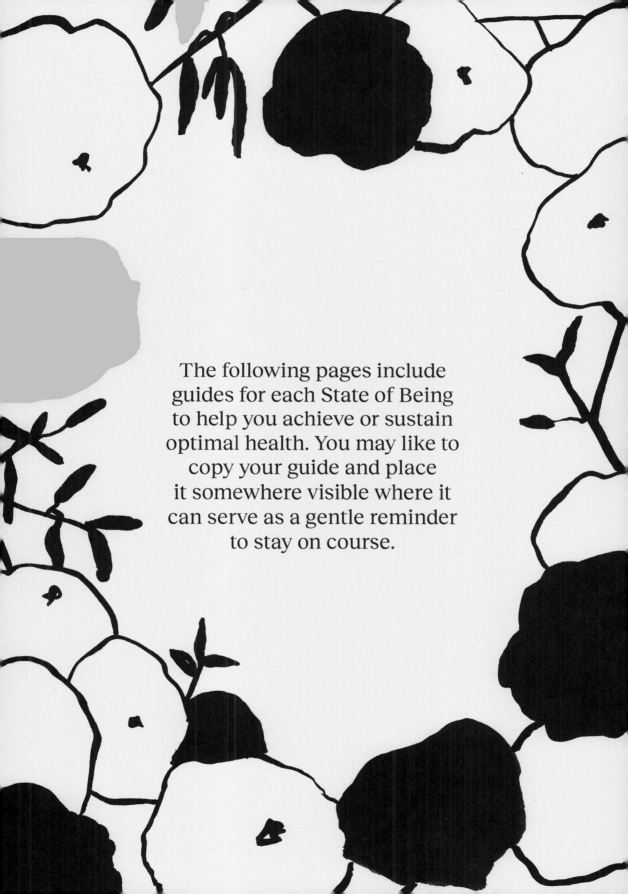

The following pages include
guides for each State of Being
to help you achieve or sustain
optimal health. You may like to
copy your guide and place
it somewhere visible where it
can serve as a gentle reminder
to stay on course.

DEPLETED STATE OF BEING

A DAILY (AND NIGHTLY) GUIDE

1   Correct your sleep hygiene. This is your first step to take before embarking on any health changes.

2   Avoid mobile phone usage for work or social media for at least two hours before sleeping and after waking.

3   Incorporate some movement – just five minutes – into your morning, within two hours of waking.

4   Try removing caffeine from your diet for a while until your body replenishes (coffee as well as black, white and green tea, and foods containing cocoa. Yes, sorry, that does mean chocolate!) Try Swiss Water-filtered decaffeinated beverages and some restorative herbal teas such as Tulsa and liquorice instead. These are wonderful supports for your adrenal glands.

5   Begin your day by gently easing yourself into your Purple Zone. Write down your tasks for the day.

6   Check your boundaries – is there something you're doing today that will deplete your energy or emotional stores? If so, address this as gently as you feel able.

7   Drink at least 1–2 litres of filtered water each day.

8 Eat for your gut. Revisit Chapter 4 for some advice. Think oily fish, nuts and plant-based dishes.

9 Reduce the amount of raw foods you are eating (such as salads) for a while to allow your gut to heal. Cooked foods are easier to digest and place less demand on your recovering digestion. Eat more cooked vegetables and nourishing foods such as hearty soups, bone broths and casseroles.

10 Sit down to enjoy your meal, especially your dinner. Make time to relax, chew your food and nourish your body. Consider foods to help you sleep and feed good gut health (see Chapter 4).

11 For a while. avoid gluten and dairy products as much as possible.

12 Moved into the Red Zone? What happened? Be as honest as possible about what you can take responsibility for, and what you can leave aside.

13 Take some time to walk and lie around in nature. This could be up to an hour of enjoying the rainforest, a park or the beach.

14 Sit and do nothing. Whether this is a meditation or time to return to the Blue Zone, this is a non-negotiable part of your day.

15 Take up something that is creative, such as knitting, cooking, sewing, writing, art, pottery or even playing a musical instrument. Think of something that you enjoy and will get lost in doing.

16 A nightly ritual is an essential part of your sleep hygiene (see Chapter 9). Perhaps take a warm bath, add some dead sea salts or magnesium salts and lavender essential oils. Maybe you would enjoy being propped up in bed reading a calming book or sitting beside the fire reading or even just watching the flames dance. It is simple repetitive rituals like this that signal to your body that it's time to sleep.

17 Sleep well.

SURVIVING STATE OF BEING

A DAILY (AND NIGHTLY) GUIDE

1   Sleep hygiene. Are there any areas of your nightime routine that could do with improvement? If so, make one change today for a better night's sleep tonight.

2   Avoid work emails and social media for at least two hours before sleeping and after waking.

3   Move your body within one hour of waking. This could be Qi Gong, yoga, Pilates, cardio interval training, walking, swimming or stretching.

4   Enjoy a healthy breakfast which includes all the food groups of carbohydrate, protein and whole fats (such as avocado and mushrooms/ eggs on sourdough bread).

5   Begin your day with some mindfulness exercises or journalling.

6   On your way to work remind yourself to be kind to you, telling yourself to remember to breathe and that you will face any challenges in your Purple Zone knowing that this is your best self to be productive.

7   Check that your boundaries are firmly in place. Be honest about any situations that may have recently occurred, or events that are planned that are making you feel anxious. How can you re-set your boundaries

in these instances? (Revisit Chapter 6 for some tips).

8 Check your Zones. If you feel yourself tipping into the Red Zone, take some time out. Go for a walk if you can, even if it is into another room or ideally out in nature. Remember to practice diaphragmatic breathing and think helpful thoughts. Design a mantra like 'this too will pass'. Slowly drink a big glass of water.

9 Your wind-down routine will set you up for restorative sleep. What could you incorporate tonight? Perhaps an aromatic bath with dead sea salts or Epsom salts with a calming essential oil such as lavender added. Try some breathing and meditation - this could be a new helpful health habit to incorporate into your sleep hygiene.

10 Sleep well.

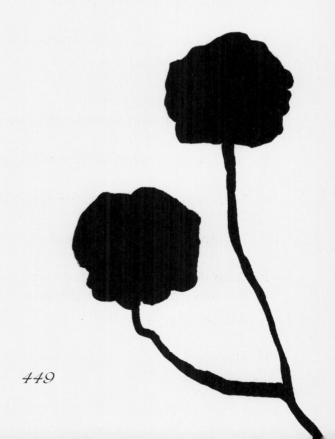

THRIVING STATE OF BEING

A DAILY (AND NIGHTLY) GUIDE

1   How did you sleep? Continuing good sleep habits will help to keep you in this State of Being.

2   Avoid work emails and social media for at least two hours before sleeping and after waking.

3   Get moving. Would your body benefit from some movement today? If so where? A change of pace can help keep you interested in exercise.

4   Journal about how you feel and what's going on with your life.

5   Tackle some tasks to help you get ahead for the week. Taking care of small business can go a long way to reducing stress in the long run.

6   Be creative! Make something with your hands, or bake. This will help you to remain relax and express yourself.

7   Head outdoors - spend some time in nature, gardening or bushwalking.

8   Batch-cook some meals to ensure you continue to eat well during the week.

9   Invite a friend or family for dinner.

10 Wind down. Meditation should be part of your daily sleep hygiene - remember to keep this good habit for a good night's sleep. A bath can provide a simple medium to ease tension for both mind and body.

11 Sleep well.

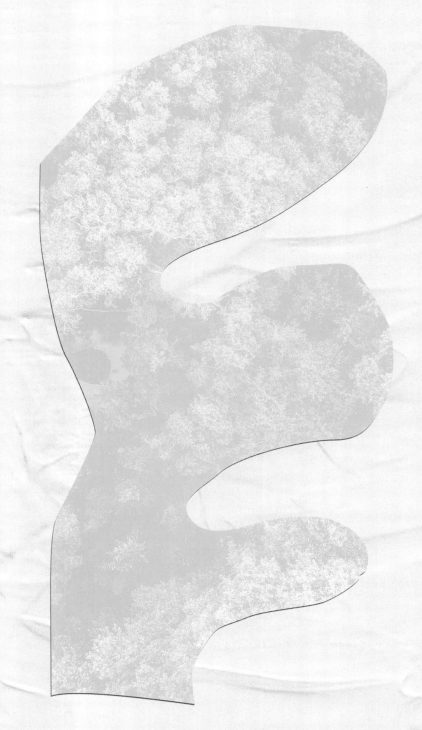

Fin. For now.

Resources

Our websites
drkaren.com.au
sharonkolkka.com.au

To confirm the qualifications, registration and to find all healthcare practitioners

The Australian Health Practitioner Regulation Agency (AHPRA)
ahpra.gov.au

Chinese medical practitioners

Chinese Medicine Board of Australia
chinesemedicineboard.com.au

Crisis care, support and suicide prevention

Lifeline
lifeline.org.au
13 11 14

Beyond Blue
beyondblue.org.au
1300 224 636

Integrative medical doctors

Australian Integrative Medical Association (AIMA)
aima.net.au

Australian College of Nutritional and Environmental Medicine (ACNEM)
acnem.org

Mental and emotional wellbeing

Psychologists
Contact your local GP for Medicare-based referral to a local psychologist.

PsychHelp
psychelp.com.au

Parent Line; free phone counselling for parents
parentline.com.au
1300 30 1300

Kids Helpline; for young people aged 5 – 25 years
kidshelpline.com.au
1800 55 1800

The Journey
Find a practitioner in your area
thejourney.com
(search your country)

Equine Assisted Therapy
esta.com.au
admin@eata.net.au (email for guidance to find a therapist in your area)

Movement practitioners

C.H.E.K Practitioners
chekconnect.com

Exercise and Sport Science Australia
essa.org.au

Registered nutritionists

Nutrition Society of Australia
nsa.asn.au

PCOS Resources

PCOS Essentials Wellness Program by Dr Karen Coates, found at
thePCOSdoctor.com

Physiotherapists And Pilates

Australian Physiotherapy Association
australian.physio

Other solutions for sleep and physical wellbeing

Workpace
wellnomics.com/workpace-download-registered-version/

SleepCycle
sleepcycle.com

For further reading, we suggest the following authors

Dr Libby Weaver
Brandon Bays
Byron Katie
Dr Daniel Siegel
Michael Pollan
Dr Deepak Chopra
Professor Brené Brown
Marshall Rosenberg
Bruce Lipton
Dan Buettner
Donna Farhi
Bill Lee-Emery

References

Chapter 1: What's Your State of Being?

1   Radostina K. Purvanova, John P. Muros, Gender differences in burnout: A meta-analysis, Journal of Vocational Behavior, Volume 77, Issue 2, 2010, Pages 168-185, ISSN 0001-8791, https://doi.org/10.1016/j.jvb.2010.04.006.

Chapter 3: Nourishment

1   Willett WC, Koplan JP, Nugent R, et al. Prevention of Chronic Disease by Means of Diet and Lifestyle Changes. In: Jamison DT, Breman JG, Measham AR, et al., editors. Disease Control Priorities in Developing Countries. 2nd edition. Washington (DC): The International Bank for Reconstruction and Development / The World Bank; 2006. Chapter 44.

2   http://media.healthdirect.org.au/publications/Nutrition-Information-Panel.pdf

3   Eating Disorder Statistics & Key Research | Eating Disorders Victoria

4   Abdel-Salam OM, Salem NA, El-Shamarka ME, Hussein JS, Ahmed NA, El-Nagar ME. Studies on the effects of aspartame on memory and oxidative stress in brain of mice. Eur Rev Med Pharmacol Sci. 2012 Dec;16(15):2092-101.

5   Krause N, Wegner A. Fructose Metabolism in Cancer. Cells. 2020 Dec 8;9(12):2635. doi: 10.3390/cells9122635. PMID: 33302403; PMCID: PMC7762580.

6   Mirtschink P, Jang C, Arany Z, Krek W. Fructose metabolism, cardiometabolic risk, and the epidemic of coronary artery disease. Eur Heart J. 2018 Jul 7;39(26):2497-2505. doi: 10.1093/eurheartj/ehx518. PMID: 29020416; PMCID: PMC6037111.

7   Viazzi F, Genovesi S, Ambruzzi MA, Giussani M. Sugar, fructose, uric acid and hypertension in children and adolescents. Ital J Pediatr. 2015 Sep 30;41(Suppl 2):A76. doi: 10.1186/1824-7288-41-S2-A76. PMCID: PMC4707621.

8   Wiss DA, Avena N, Rada P. Sugar Addiction: From Evolution to Revolution. Front Psychiatry. 2018 Nov 7;9:545. doi: 10.3389/fpsyt.2018.00545. PMID: 30464748; PMCID: PMC6234835.

9   Eric Robinson, Paul Aveyard, Amanda Daley, Kate Jolly, Amanda Lewis, Deborah Lycett, Suzanne Higgs, Eating attentively: a systematic review and meta-analysis of the effect of food intake memory and awareness on eating, The American Journal of Clinical Nutrition, Volume 97, Issue 4, April 2013, Pages 728–742, https://doi.org/10.3945/ajcn.112.045245

10 Eric Robinson, Paul Aveyard, Amanda Daley, Kate Jolly, Amanda Lewis, Deborah Lycett, Suzanne Higgs, Eating attentively: a systematic review and meta-analysis of the effect of food intake memory and awareness on eating, The American Journal of Clinical Nutrition, Volume 97, Issue 4, April 2013, Pages 728–742, https://doi.org/10.3945/ajcn.112.045245

11 https://www.heartfoundation.org.au/Blog/DRAFT-Sorting-fat-from-fiction

12 Ramsden C E, Zamora D, Majchrzak-Hong S, Faurot K R, Broste S K, Frantz R P et al. Re-evaluation of the traditional diet-heart hypothesis: analysis of recovered data from Minnesota Coronary Experiment (1968-73) BMJ 2016; 353 :i1246

13 Aune D, Giovannucci E, Boffetta P, Fadnes LT, Keum N, Norat T, Greenwood DC, Riboli E, Vatten LJ, Tonstad S. Fruit and vegetable intake and the risk of cardiovascular disease, total cancer and all-cause mortality-a systematic review and dose-response meta-analysis of prospective studies. Int J Epidemiol. 2017 Jun 1;46(3):1029-1056. doi: 10.1093/ije/dyw319. PMID: 28338764; PMCID: PMC5837313.

Chapter 4: You and Your Gut

1 Mathieu C, Duval R, Xu X, Rodrigues-Lima F, Dupret JM. Effects of pesticide chemicals on the activity of metabolic enzymes: focus on thiocarbamates. Expert Opin Drug Metab Toxicol. 2015 Jan;11(1):81-94. doi: 10.1517/17425255.2015.975691. Epub 2014 Nov 13. PMID: 25391334.

2 Lăcătuşu CM, Grigorescu ED, Floria M, Onofriescu A, Mihai BM. The Mediterranean Diet: From an Environment-Driven Food Culture to an Emerging Medical Prescription. Int J Environ Res Public Health. 2019 Mar 15;16(6):942. doi: 10.3390/ijerph16060942. PMID: 30875998; PMCID: PMC6466433.

3 https://www.healthline.com/health-news/does-80-20-diet-actually-help-you-lose-weight

4 Terciolo C, Dapoigny M, Andre F. Beneficial effects of Saccharomyces boulardii CNCM I-745 on clinical disorders associated with intestinal barrier disruption. Clin Exp Gastroenterol. 2019 Feb 11;12:67-82. doi: 10.2147/CEG.S181590. PMID: 30804678; PMCID: PMC6375115.

5 Jothimani D, Kailasam E, Danielraj S, Nallathambi B, Ramachandran H, Sekar P, Manoharan S, Ramani V, Narasimhan G, Kaliamoorthy I, Rela M. COVID-19: Poor outcomes in patients with zinc deficiency. Int J Infect Dis. 2020 Nov;100:343-349. doi: 10.1016/j.ijid.2020.09.014. Epub 2020 Sep 10. PMID: 32920234; PMCID: PMC7482607.

6 Zinc | COVID-19 Treatment Guidelines (nih.gov)

Chapter 5: Functional Movement and Exercise

1 Chaput JP, Carson V, Gray CE, Tremblay MS. Importance of all movement behaviors in a 24 hour period for overall health. Int J Environ Res Public Health. 2014 Dec 4;11(12):12575-81. doi: 10.3390/ijerph111212575. PMID: 25485978; PMCID: PMC4276632.

2 American College of Cardiology. "Couch potatoes beware: Too much time spent watching TV is harmful to heart health." ScienceDaily. ScienceDaily, 11 January 2011.

3 Scofield KL, Hecht S. Bone health in endurance athletes: runners, cyclists, and swimmers. Curr Sports Med Rep. 2012 Nov-Dec;11(6):328-34. doi: 10.1249/JSR.0b013e3182779193. PMID: 23147022.

4 Śliwicka E, Cisoń T, Pilaczyńska-Szcześniak Ł, Ziemba A, Straburzyńska-Lupa A. Effects of marathon race on selected myokines and sclerostin in middle-aged male amateur runners. Sci Rep. 2021 Feb 2;11(1):2813. doi: 10.1038/s41598-021-82288-z. PMID: 33531538; PMCID: PMC7854637.

5 Rogers MA, Evans WJ. Changes in skeletal muscle with aging: effects of exercise training. Exerc Sport Sci Rev. 1993;21:65-102. PMID: 8504850.

6 Ekelund U, Steene-Johannessen J, Brown WJ, Fagerland MW, Owen N, Powell KE, Bauman A, Lee IM; Lancet Physical Activity Series 2 Executive Committe; Lancet Sedentary Behaviour Working Group. Does physical activity attenuate, or even eliminate, the detrimental association of sitting time with mortality? A harmonised meta-analysis of data from more than 1 million men and women. Lancet. 2016 Sep 24;388(10051):1302-10. doi: 10.1016/S0140-6736(16)30370-1. Epub 2016 Jul 28. Erratum in: Lancet. 2016 Sep 24;388(10051):e6. PMID: 27475271.

7 Andersen LB, Mota J, Di Pietro L. Update on the global pandemic of physical inactivity. Lancet. 2016 Sep 24;388(10051):1255-6. doi: 10.1016/S0140-6736(16)30960-6. Epub 2016 Jul 28. PMID: 27475275.

8 Sisson SB, Camhi SM, Church TS, Martin CK, Tudor-Locke C, Bouchard C, Earnest CP, Smith SR, Newton RL Jr, Rankinen T, Katzmarzyk PT. Leisure time sedentary behavior, occupational/domestic physical activity, and metabolic syndrome in U.S. men and women. Metab Syndr Relat Disord. 2009 Dec;7(6):529-36. doi: 10.1089/met.2009.0023. PMID: 19900152; PMCID: PMC2796695.

9 van der Ploeg HP, Chey T, Korda RJ, Banks E, Bauman A. Sitting time and all-cause mortality risk in 222 497 Australian adults. Arch Intern Med. 2012 Mar 26;172(6):494-500. doi: 10.1001/archinternmed.2011.2174. PMID: 22450936.

Chapter 6: Emotional Wellbeing

1   *Aimee M. Hunter, Ian A. Cook, Andrew F. Leuchter. Does prior antidepressant treatment of major depression impact brain function during current treatment? European Neuropsychopharmacology, 2012; DOI:* **10.1016/j.euroneuro.2012.02.005**

2   *https://www.campaigntoendloneliness.org/the-facts-on-loneliness/*

3   *https://greatergood.berkeley.edu/article/item/the_new_science_of_forgiveness*

4   *https://www.aihw.gov.au/reports/life-expectancy-death/deaths-in-australia/contents/leading-causes-of-death*

5   https://www.researchgate.net/publication/233120784_Ethnic_habitus_and_young_children_a_case_study_of_Northern_Ireland

6   *The psychology of religion and coping: theory, research, practice Kenneth Pargament Gilford Press 2001*

7   *Anderson CL, Monroy M, Keltner D. Awe in nature heals: Evidence from military veterans, at-risk youth, and college students. Emotion. 2018 Dec;18(8):1195-1202. doi: 10.1037/emo0000442. Epub 2018 Jun 21. PMID: 29927260.*

8   *Willett WC, Koplan JP, Nugent R, et al. Prevention of Chronic Disease by Means of Diet and Lifestyle Changes. In: Jamison DT, Breman JG, Measham AR, et al., editors. Disease Control Priorities in Developing Countries. 2nd edition. Washington (DC): The International Bank for Reconstruction and Development / The World Bank; 2006. Chapter 44.*

9   *GBD 2016 Alcohol Collaborators. Alcohol use and burden for 195 countries and territories, 1990-2016: a systematic analysis for the Global Burden of Disease Study 2016. Lancet. 2018 Sep 22;392(10152):1015-1035. doi: 10.1016/S0140-6736(18)31310-2. Epub 2018 Aug 23. PMID: 30146330; PMCID: PMC6148333.*

Chapter 9: Sleep

1   *Berger M, Gray JA, Roth BL. The expanded biology of serotonin. Annu Rev Med. 2009;60:355-66. doi: 10.1146/annurev.med.60.042307.110802. PMID: 19630576; PMCID: PMC5864293.*

2   *Institute of Medicine (US) Committee on Sleep Medicine and Research; Colten HR, Altevogt BM, editors. Sleep Disorders and Sleep Deprivation: An Unmet Public Health Problem. Washington (DC): National Academies Press (US); 2006. 3, Extent and Health Consequences of Chronic Sleep Loss and Sleep Disorders. Available from: https://www.ncbi.nlm.nih.gov/books/NBK19961/*

3   *Prather AA, Leung CW, Adler NE, Ritchie L, Laraia B, Epel ES. Short and sweet: Associations between self-reported sleep duration and sugar-sweetened beverage consumption among adults in the United States. Sleep Health. 2016 Dec;2(4):272-276. doi: 10.1016/j.sleh.2016.09.007. PMID: 28393097; PMCID: PMC5380400.*

4   *Costa G. Shift work and health: current problems and preventive actions. Saf Health Work. 2010 Dec;1(2):112-23. doi: 10.5491/SHAW.2010.1.2.112. Epub 2010 Dec 30. PMID: 22953171; PMCID: PMC3430894.*

5   *Meng X, Li Y, Li S, Zhou Y, Gan RY, Xu DP, Li HB. Dietary Sources and Bioactivities of Melatonin. Nutrients. 2017 Apr 7;9(4):367. doi: 10.3390/nu9040367. PMID: 28387721; PMCID: PMC5409706.*

6   *Maroo N, Hazra A, Das T. Efficacy and safety of a polyherbal sedative-hypnotic formulation NSF-3 in primary insomnia in comparison to zolpidem: a randomized controlled trial. Indian J Pharmacol. 2013 Jan-Feb;45(1):34-9. doi: 10.4103/0253-7613.106432. PMID: 23543804; PMCID: PMC3608291.*

Chapter 10: Thriving in a Toxic World

1 *Crain, AD, Janssen, S. et al. Female reproductive disorders: The roles of endocrine disrupting compounds and developmental timing. Fertility and Sterility; expected publication Fall 2008.*

2 *Janda K, Jakubczyk K, Baranowska-Bosiacka I, Kapczuk P, Kochman J, Rębacz-Maron E, Gutowska I. Mineral Composition and Antioxidant Potential of Coffee Beverages Depending on the Brewing Method. Foods. 2020 Jan 23;9(2):121. doi: 10.3390/foods9020121. PMID: 31979386; PMCID: PMC7074357.*

3 *Kwang Jin Kim et al. Efficiency of Volatile Formaldehyde Removal by Indoor Plants: Contribution of Aerial Plant Parts versus the Root Zone. Horticultural Science, 133: 479-627 (2008)*

4 *Mariana M, Feiteiro J, Verde I, Cairrao E. The effects of phthalates in the cardiovascular and reproductive systems: A review. Environ Int. 2016 Sep;94:758-776. doi: 10.1016/j.envint.2016.07.004. PMID: 27424259.*

5 *Mariana M, Cairrao E. Phthalates Implications in the Cardiovascular System. J Cardiovasc Dev Dis. 2020 Jul 22;7(3):26. doi: 10.3390/jcdd7030026. PMID: 32707888; PMCID: PMC7570088.*

6 *Chu PC, Wu C, Su TC. Association between Urinary Phthalate Metabolites and Markers of Endothelial Dysfunction in Adolescents and Young Adults. Toxics. 2021 Feb 6;9(2):33. doi: 10.3390/toxics9020033. PMID: 33562063; PMCID: PMC7915273.*

7 *Heudorf U, Mersch-Sundermann V, Angerer J. Phthalates: toxicology and exposure. Int J Hyg Environ Health. 2007 Oct;210(5):623-34. doi: 10.1016/j.ijheh.2007.07.011. Epub 2007 Sep 21. PMID: 17889607.*

Chapter 11: Secret Women's Business – Finding Hormonal Harmony

1 *https://www.unicef.org.au/blog/stories/may-2019/800-million*

2 *https://www.jeanhailes.org.au/health-a-z/periods/premenstrual-syndrome-pms*

3 *journals.sagepub.com/doi/pdf/10.1177/216507990104900203*

4 https://www.jeanhailes.org.au/health-a-z/periods/premenstrual-syndrome-pms

5 *Victoria H Stiles, Brad S Metcalf, Karen M Knapp, Alex V Rowlands. A small amount of precisely measured high-intensity habitual physical activity predicts bone health in pre- and post-menopausal women in UK Biobank. International Journal of Epidemiology, 2017; DOI: 10.1093/ije/dyx080*

6 *Dunn RR, Amato KR, Archie EA, Arandjelovic M, Crittenden AN and Nichols LM (2020) The Internal, External and Extended Microbiomes of Hominins. Front. Ecol. Evol. 8:25. doi: 10.3389/fevo.2020.00025*

Chapter 12: Nutrigenomics

1 *Soubry A, Hoyo C, Jirtle RL, Murphy SK. A paternal environmental legacy: evidence for epigenetic inheritance through the male germ line. Bioessays. 2014 Apr;36(4):359-71. doi: 10.1002/bies.201300113. Epub 2014 Jan 16. PMID: 24431278; PMCID: PMC4047566.*

Index

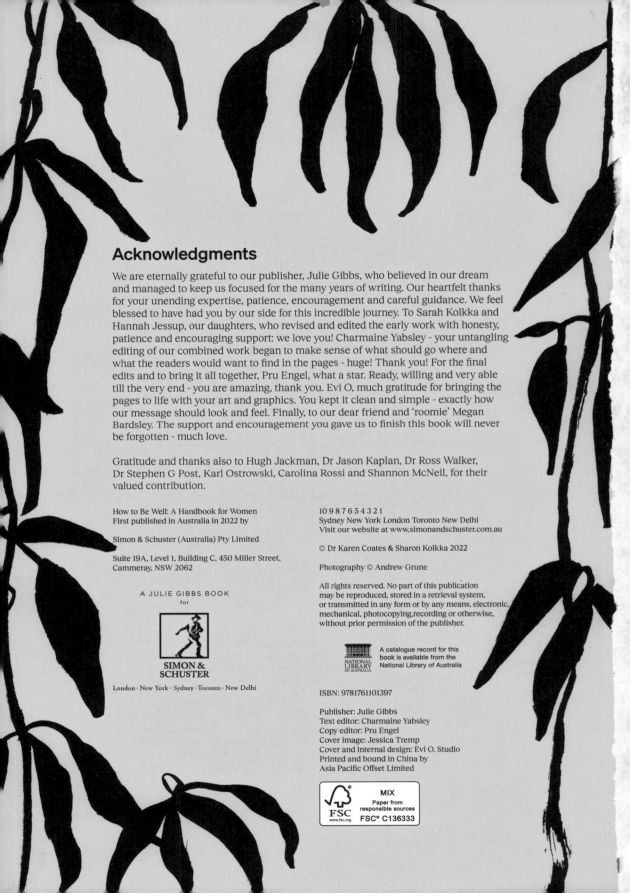

Acknowledgments

We are eternally grateful to our publisher, Julie Gibbs, who believed in our dream and managed to keep us focused for the many years of writing. Our heartfelt thanks for your unending expertise, patience, encouragement and careful guidance. We feel blessed to have had you by our side for this incredible journey. To Sarah Kolkka and Hannah Jessup, our daughters, who revised and edited the early work with honesty, patience and encouraging support: we love you! Charmaine Yabsley - your untangling editing of our combined work began to make sense of what should go where and what the readers would want to find in the pages - huge! Thank you! For the final edits and to bring it all together, Pru Engel, what a star. Ready, willing and very able till the very end - you are amazing, thank you. Evi O, much gratitude for bringing the pages to life with your art and graphics. You kept it clean and simple - exactly how our message should look and feel. Finally, to our dear friend and 'roomie' Megan Bardsley. The support and encouragement you gave us to finish this book will never be forgotten - much love.

Gratitude and thanks also to Hugh Jackman, Dr Jason Kaplan, Dr Ross Walker, Dr Stephen G Post, Karl Ostrowski, Carolina Rossi and Shannon McNeil, for their valued contribution.

How to Be Well: A Handbook for Women
First published in Australia in 2022 by

Simon & Schuster (Australia) Pty Limited

Suite 19A, Level 1, Building C, 450 Miller Street,
Cammeray, NSW 2062

A JULIE GIBBS BOOK
for

**SIMON &
SCHUSTER**

London · New York · Sydney · Toronto · New Delhi

10 9 8 7 6 5 4 3 2 1
Sydney New York London Toronto New Delhi
Visit our website at www.simonandschuster.com.au

© Dr Karen Coates & Sharon Kolkka 2022

Photography © Andrew Grune

All rights reserved. No part of this publication may be reproduced, stored in a retrieval system, or transmitted in any form or by any means, electronic, mechanical, photocopying, recording or otherwise, without prior permission of the publisher.

A catalogue record for this book is available from the National Library of Australia

ISBN: 9781761101397

Publisher: Julie Gibbs
Text editor: Charmaine Yabsley
Copy editor: Pru Engel
Cover image: Jessica Tremp
Cover and internal design: Evi O. Studio
Printed and bound in China by
Asia Pacific Offset Limited

FSC
www.fsc.org

MIX
Paper from
responsible sources
FSC® C136333

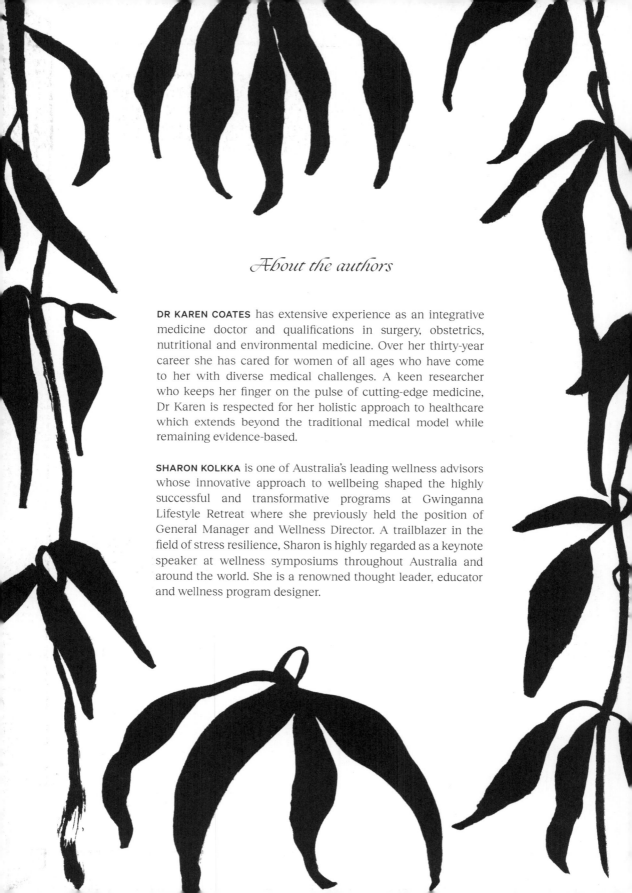

About the authors

DR KAREN COATES has extensive experience as an integrative medicine doctor and qualifications in surgery, obstetrics, nutritional and environmental medicine. Over her thirty-year career she has cared for women of all ages who have come to her with diverse medical challenges. A keen researcher who keeps her finger on the pulse of cutting-edge medicine, Dr Karen is respected for her holistic approach to healthcare which extends beyond the traditional medical model while remaining evidence-based.

SHARON KOLKKA is one of Australia's leading wellness advisors whose innovative approach to wellbeing shaped the highly successful and transformative programs at Gwinganna Lifestyle Retreat where she previously held the position of General Manager and Wellness Director. A trailblazer in the field of stress resilience, Sharon is highly regarded as a keynote speaker at wellness symposiums throughout Australia and around the world. She is a renowned thought leader, educator and wellness program designer.